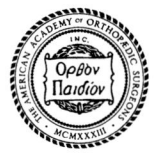

American Academy of Orthopaedic Surgeons
6300 North River Road
Rosemont, Illinois 60018
1-800-626-6726

The Unstable Shoulder

EDITED BY
LOUIS U. BIGLIANI, MD
Chief, The Shoulder Service
Vice-Chairman, Department of Orthopaedic Surgery
New York Orthopaedic Hospital
Columbia Presbyterian Medical Center
New York, New York

CONTRIBUTORS
LTC Robert A. Arciero, MD
Evan L. Flatow, MD
Roger G. Pollock, MD
James E. Tibone, MD
Jon J.P. Warner, MD

SERIES EDITOR
Glenn B. Pfeffer, MD

American Academy of Orthopaedic Surgeons

THE UNSTABLE SHOULDER

Director, Department of Publications
Marilyn L. Fox, PhD

Senior Editor
Bruce Davis

Associate Senior Editor
Jane Baque

Production Manager
Loraine Edwalds

Graphic Design Coordinator
Pamela Hutton Erickson

Editorial Assistants
Brigid Flanagan
Sophie Tosta

Production Assistant
Jana Ronayne

Publications Secretary
Geraldine Dubberke

The American Academy of Orthopaedic Surgeons Monograph Series is dedicated to Wendy O. Schmidt, American Academy of Orthopaedic Surgeons senior medical editor, 1987-1991.

The Unstable Shoulder
edited by Louis U. Bigliani, MD

ISBN 0-89203-120-4

CONTENTS

CONTRIBUTORS

LTC Robert A. Arciero, MD
Head Team Physician
United States Military Academy
West Point, New York

Louis U. Bigliani, MD
Chief, The Shoulder Service
Vice-Chairman, Department of
  Orthopaedic Surgery
New York Orthopaedic Hospital
Columbia-Presbyterian Medical Center
New York, New York

Evan L. Flatow, MD
Herbert Irving Associate Professor of
  Orthopaedic Surgery
Associate Chief, The Shoulder Service
New York Orthopaedic Hospital
Columbia-Presbyterian Medical Center
New York, New York

Roger G. Pollock, MD
Assistant Professor of Orthopaedic Surgery
Columbia University
Assistant Attending, The Shoulder Service
Columbia-Presbyterian Medical Center
New York, New York

James E. Tibone, MD
Clinical Professor, Department of Orthopaedics
University of Southern California
Associate, Kerlan-Jobe Orthopaedic Clinic
Inglewood, California

Jon J.P. Warner, MD
Director, The Shoulder Service
Assistant Professor, Department of
  Orthopaedic Surgery
University of Pittsburgh
Pittsburgh, Pennsylvania

PREFACE

Glenohumeral instability is one of the most complex and challenging areas of shoulder pathology to diagnose and treat. It also has been one of the oldest areas of shoulder interest, capturing the attention of the ancient Greeks more than 2,000 years ago as they struggled with different diagnostic and treatment problems. Interestingly enough, many of the same dilemmas and problems trouble us today in our management of shoulder instability.

We are fortunate in this monograph to have an outstanding group of contributing authors who are experts in the field of shoulder instability. They have spent a great deal of time and effort to compile an excellent monograph, which includes current and relevant knowledge about the etiology, diagnosis, and treatment of shoulder instability. Every aspect of shoulder instability is addressed in a very informative manner with pertinent references for further investigation.

We hope that this monograph will help you in your practice of shoulder surgery. I would like to thank the authors and their staff for the time and effort that they have expended to make this such a worthwhile volume.

I would also like to thank Marilyn Fox, PhD, Director of the Department of Publications; Jane Baque, Joan Abern, and Bruce Davis, who managed the project and edited the manuscripts; Loraine Edwalds, who oversaw the production process; and Pamela Hutton Erickson who developed the new design for the monograph series. I would also like to acknowledge the efforts of Susan Baim, Brigid Flanagan, and Sophie Tosta, editorial assistants, Jana Ronayne, production assistant, and Geraldine Dubberke, publications secretary.

LOUIS U. BIGLIANI, MD

ANATOMY AND BIOMECHANICS

JON J.P. WARNER, MD AND EVAN L. FLATOW, MD

INTRODUCTION

Historically, the clinician's understanding of shoulder instability has been based on anecdotal, qualitative clinical experience and observations of pathology.[1-25] More recently, clinical approaches have been based on quantitative anatomic and biomechanical data resulting from a collaboration among surgeons, biomechanical engineers, anatomists, biochemists, and other basic scientists. The results of these studies have provided a clearer understanding of the unique anatomic arrangement of the glenohumeral joint as a minimally constrained articulation that permits a wide range of normal shoulder motion while balancing mobility and stability. It is this anatomic arrangement that renders the glenohumeral joint at risk for clinical instability.

RISK FACTORS FOR INSTABILITY

There is considerable individual variation in capsuloligamentous anatomy,[7,26-32] inherent "normal" shoulder laxity,[33-36] and conditioning and strength of the rotator cuff and biceps.[37] Proprioception[38-40] and scapulothoracic motion[41-43] also may play a role in shoulder stability.

Laxity is asymptomatic, passive translation of the humeral head on the glenoid that is unassociated with pain. Laxity is present to varying degrees in normal shoulders[26-29,33-35,37,44-48] and is required for normal, unrestricted glenohumeral rotation. The degree of laxity may be affected by age,[36] gender, and congenital factors.[49] Some clinicians have suggested that laxity is a risk factor for the development of clinical instability.[49,50]

Instability is a pathologic condition that is manifest as pain in association with excessive translation of the humeral head on the glenoid during active shoulder motion. There are varying degrees of instability, including subluxation and

dislocation. The primary direction of such pathologic motion may be anterior, posterior, or inferior, or a combination of directions. These descriptions are discussed in further detail under *Classification and Evaluation*.

Static and dynamic factors (capsuloligamentous structures and rotator cuff/biceps muscle action, respectively) play complex and cooperative roles in maintaining joint stability (Outline 1). No single factor is responsible for glenohumeral joint stability and no single pathology or lesion causes clinical instability (Table 1). Moreover, these factors can be modified by age, exposure to trauma, congenital anatomic variations, and muscle function.

The glenohumeral ligaments stabilize the humeral head in the glenoid in a "load-sharing" fashion. Therefore, an injury to one portion of the capsule may increase translation of the humeral head in more than one direction. Furthermore, the contribution that static and dynamic factors make to stability depends on arm position and direction of an applied force.

The shoulder can be subjected to significant levels of stress, depending on specific activities and sports participation. For example, a pitcher may subject the soft tissues of the shoulder to

TABLE 1

NORMAL AND ABNORMAL ANATOMY AND BIOMECHANICS

Stability Factor	Pathologic Condition
Glenoid version	Congenital: Abnormal version; dysplasia Fracture causing abnormal version
Humeral version	Congenital: Abnormal version; dysplasia Fracture/surgery causing abnormal version
Articular congruity	Congenital: dysplasia Acquired: fracture, Bankart lesion; wear from osteoarthritis Large Hill-Sachs lesion
Labrum	Bankart lesion "Fraying" secondary to laxity
Capsuloligamentous	Traumatic tear cumulative microtrauma causing plastic deformation Congenital laxity (possible risk factor) Loss of proprioceptive feedback
Negative intra-articular pressure	Capsular tear "Rotator interval" defect Lax capsule
Rotator cuff deficiency	Traumatic tear microtrauma (eccentric) Failure Voluntary instability
Biceps	SLAP lesion Tendon rupture
Scapulothoracic motion	Dyskinesis: fatigue and weakness of serratus long thoracic nerve palsy

repetitive, submaximal stress, which, cumulatively, can injure the capsule and ligaments. A football player may develop instability from a sudden forceful injury that ruptures or avulses the anterior capsule during a tackle.

The probability of developing clinical instability is directly related to the level of risk activity and inversely related to the quality of the static stabilizers and strength and conditioning of the dynamic stabilizers. Therefore, an individual with congenital capsular laxity or one with poorly conditioned rotator cuff muscles might theoretically be at greater risk for glenohumeral instability, especially if the activity were an overhead sport that caused repetitive submaximal loads to the glenohumeral ligaments.[51-53] Conversely, even an individual with well-developed ligaments and well-conditioned rotator cuff muscles might sustain a traumatic dislocation from a sudden force to the shoulder that exceeded the ultimate failure strength of these soft-tissue structures.

The high rate of recurrent instability after a traumatic dislocation in a younger individual is believed to result when the Bankart lesion (avulsion of the labrum) fails to heal.[9,19-23,54-57] Although this clinical impression has not been validated experimentally, capsular injury often accompanies the Bankart lesion and must be considered in a surgical approach.[26,51,58,59] The recurrence rate is believed to be lower in older individuals because capsular injuries or bony avulsions of the greater tuberosity, which are more common in this population, heal.[9,11-13,54,60-64]

STATIC FACTORS

GLENOID VERSION

In an adducted position, with the arm hanging at the side, the scapula faces 30° anteriorly on the chest wall. It is also tilted 3° upward relative to the transverse plane and 20° forward relative to the sagittal plane (Fig. 1).[32] Saha and others[65-77] have described both normal and abnormal parameters of glenoid version. In general, the glenoid averages a superior tilt of 5° and has a range of version in the transverse plane from 7° retroversion to 10° anteversion (Fig. 2). However, a wide range of variability exists and the contribution of this factor to instability remains controversial. Some surgeons[70,72,74] believe that abnormal retroversion can be a major contributing factor to posterior instability, while others[73,77] do not think that it is an important anatomic issue. The problem with these anatomic studies has been that different techniques have been used to measure glenoid version, and some of the radiographic reference axes used to measure have not been reproducible. Furthermore, Randelli and Gambrioli[77] showed that the degree of version may vary on a computed tomography (CT) scan, depending on the level of image measured.

Clinically, excessive glenoid version as a primary contributing factor to instability is probably limited to infrequent cases of posterior instability. In some rare cases this probably represents a variant of glenoid dysplasia, with the posterior portion of the glenoid failing to develop properly (Fig. 3). In most cases, excessive glenoid retroversion or anteversion is probably acquired from eccentric cartilage and bony wear in cases of arthritis. In these cases, if the humeral head is to be recentered on the glenoid by a surgical procedure, normal glenoid version should be restored in addition to any soft-tissue procedures.

HUMERAL VERSION

The articular surface of the humeral head is inclined dorsally and in retrotorsion relative to its shaft. The neck-shaft angle averages 130° to 140°, and retrotorsion averages 30° relative to the

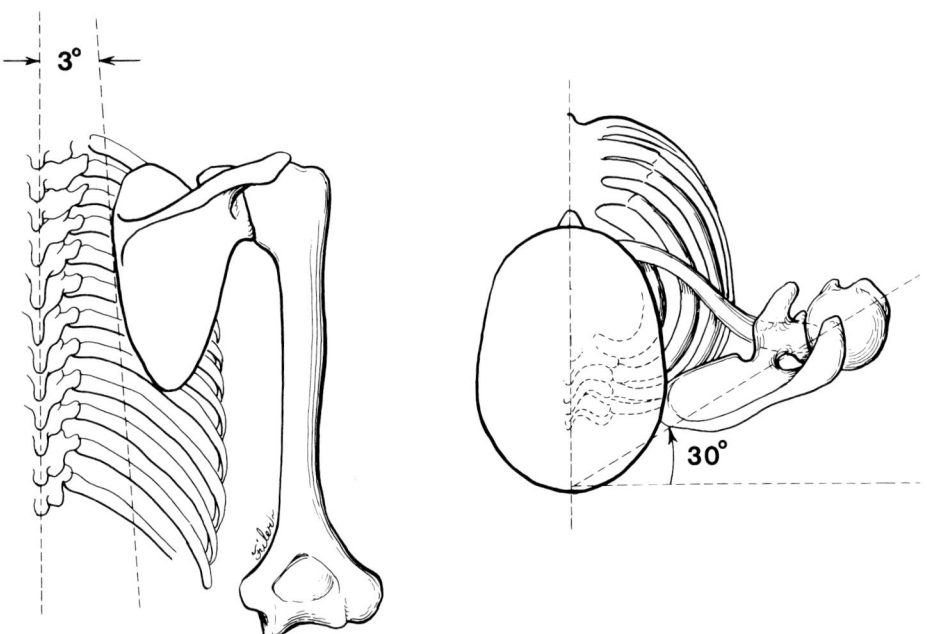

FIGURE 1
Position of the scapula on the chest wall (see text). (Reproduced with permission from Warner JJP: The gross anatomy of the joint surfaces, ligaments, labrum, and capsule, in Matsen FA III, Fu FH, Hawkins RJ (eds): *The Shoulder: A Balance of Mobility and Stability*. Rosemont, IL, American Academy of Orthopaedic Surgeons, 1993, pp 7-27.)

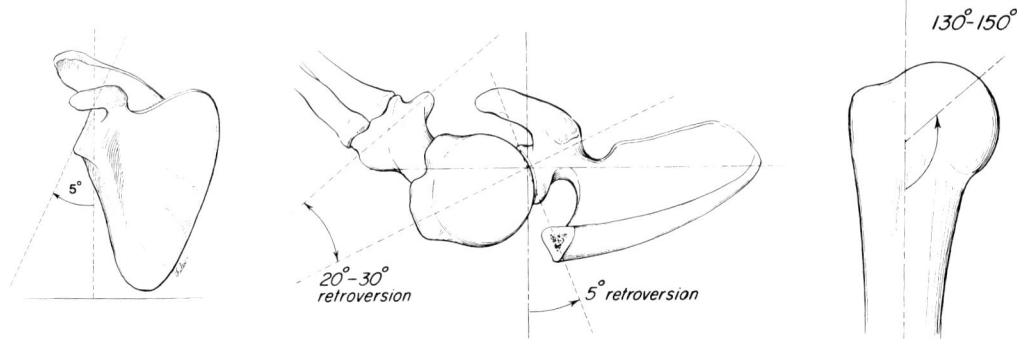

FIGURE 2

Left, Superior tilt of the glenoid (see text). (Reproduced with permission from Warner JJP: The gross anatomy of the joint surfaces, ligaments, labrum, and capsule, in Matsen FA III, Fu FH, Hawkins RJ (eds): *The Shoulder: A Balance of Mobility and Stability.* Rosemont, IL, American Academy of Orthopaedic Surgeons, 1993, pp 7-27.) **Center** and **right,** Glenoid and humeral version, and neck-shaft angle of the proximal humerus (see text). (Reproduced with permission from Warner JJP, Caborn DNM: Overview of shoulder instability. *Crit Rev Phys Rehab Med* 1992;4:145-198.)

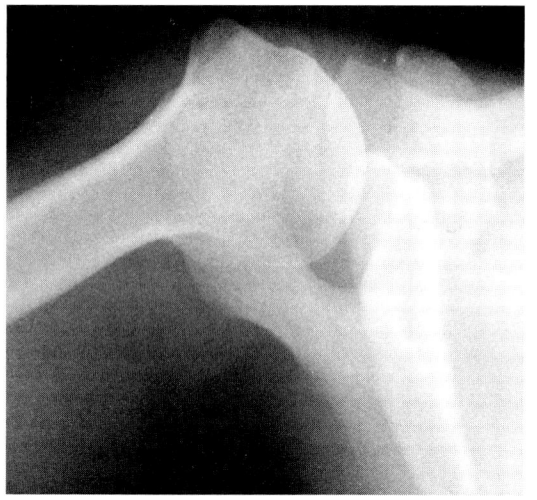 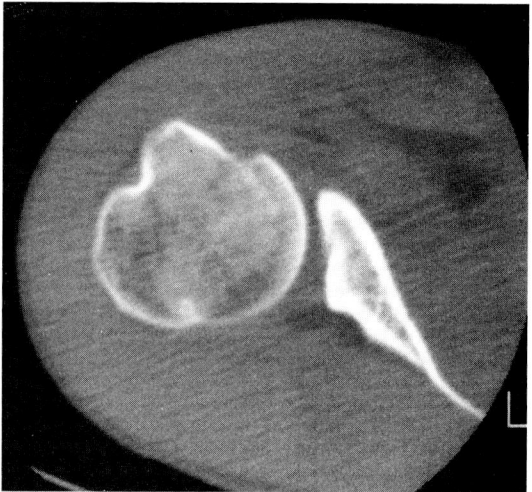

FIGURE 3

Left, Axillary radiograph of patient with glenoid hypoplasia showing excessive retroversion. **Right,** Computed tomography scan of patient with glenoid hypoplasia and retroversion.

transepicondylar axis of the distal humerus (Fig. 2, *right*).[66,67,77,78] Kronberg and associates[79,80] used radiographic measurements to demonstrate that there was significantly less humeral retrotorsion in shoulders of individuals with recurrent anterior instability (26°±4°) compared to volunteers with normal shoulders (33°±9°). Although some European surgeons have suggested using rotational osteotomy of the humerus to treat insta-

bility,[71,79-85] this is not a generally practiced approach in North America. Abnormal humeral torsion is often the result of either fracture malunion or developmental anomalies.

ARTICULAR CONFORMITY

The glenoid surface is shaped like an inverted comma, with a narrow superior area and a broader inferior area. The average vertical and trans-

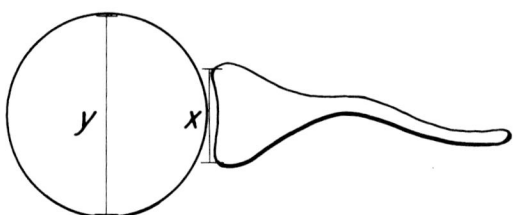

FIGURE 4

Surface area mismatch of the humeral head (y) and the glenoid (x) articular surfaces (see text). (Reproduced with permission from Warner JJP, Caborn DNM: Overview of shoulder instability. *Crit Rev Phys Rehab Med* 1992; 4:145-198.)

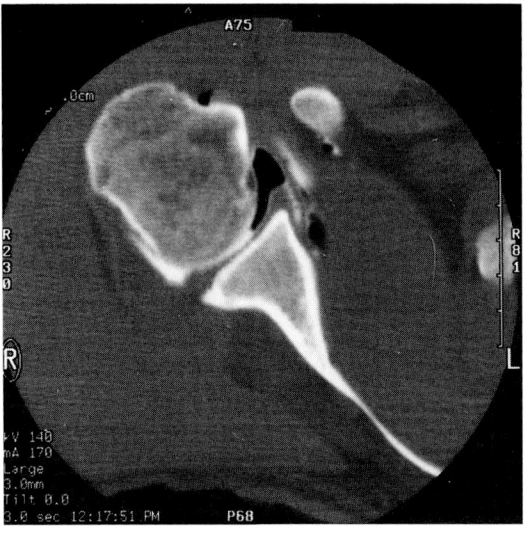

FIGURE 5

Computed tomography scan with air and contrast shows that the articular (cartilaginous) surfaces are closely conforming, although the bony glenoid appears flat.

verse dimensions of the glenoid are 35 mm and 25 mm, respectively, compared to the larger humeral head, which has vertical and transverse dimensions averaging 48 mm and 45 mm, respectively.[32] This surface area mismatch is expressed as a glenohumeral index (GH$_I$):

$$GH_I = \frac{\text{Maximum glenoid diameter}}{\text{Maximum humeral head diameter}}$$

Saha[66,67] and others[27,45] have determined that the GH$_I$ averages 0.75 and 0.76 in the sagittal and transverse planes, respectively. This size mismatch of the humeral head on the glenoid has been compared to a golf ball sitting on a tee or a basketball in a teacup (Fig. 4).[19]

Historically, articular geometry was always believed to be less important than soft-tissue factors in stabilizing the glenohumeral joint. This was justified by citing the small area of the glenoid compared to the humeral head and by the belief that the glenoid had a radius of curvature smaller than the humeral head.[66,67] The articular surfaces of the humeral head and glenoid, however, are almost perfectly matched, with a congruence to within 3 mm.[52,86] Plain radiographs can give the impression that the glenoid surface is flatter than the humeral head articular surface; however, magnetic resonance imaging (MRI) or CT that shows the cartilage surfaces demonstrate how closely the concavity of the glenoid matches the humeral head convexity (Fig. 5). As would be expected in a conforming joint, one study of glenohumeral contact using an optical, noninvasive stereophotogrammetric technique showed fairly uniform contact over the glenoid surface.[87] Another study using interposed pressure-sensitive film, however,

showed less even contact and suggested that the glenoid-humeral fit is more conformed in abduction than adduction.[88] A perfect match of the humeral head in the glenoid would be expected to result in ball-and-socket configuration. Although studies of passive glenohumeral motion have suggested that some coupled translation may accompany glenohumeral rotations,[33-35] a study of glenohumeral kinematics with simulated muscle forces very nearly showed ball-in-socket motion.[89] In contrast to previous studies,[90] this study also assessed translation by tracking the geometric center of the actual (cartilage) articular surface rather than the center of the subchondral bone as seen on radiographs. Thus, surface area mismatch is probably more important as a predisposing factor for instability than articular incongruency. An example would be any condition that disrupts the normal congruent fit and surface area relationship of the glenohumeral joint. Two examples are glenoid dysplasia and glenoid fracture (Figs. 3 and 6).[19,22,91-100]

Humeral surface loss seems less important. The Hill-Sachs lesion is an impression fracture of the posterolateral margin of the humeral head created when it dislocates over the anterior glenoid rim.[6,8,101-103] This lesion is present in more than 80% of anterior dislocations and 25% of anterior subluxations;[104] it is larger with dislocations

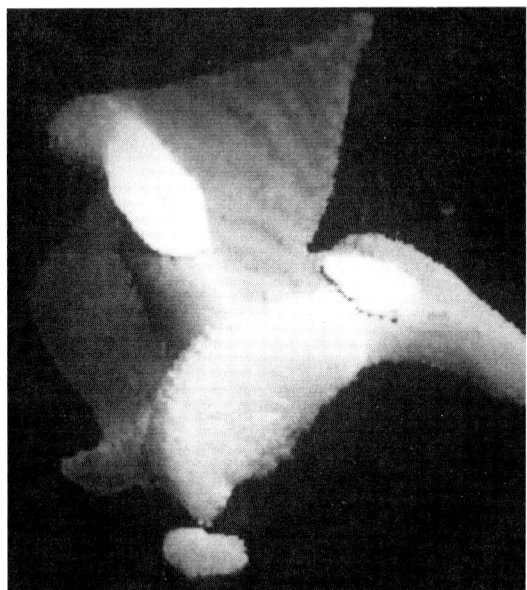

FIGURE 6
A three-dimensional computed tomography scan of a patient with loss of the anterior one third of the glenoid due to fracture. (Reproduced with permission from Warner JJP, Marks PH: Managment of complications of surgery for anterior shoulder instability. *Sports Med Arthroscopy Rev* 1993;1:272-292.)

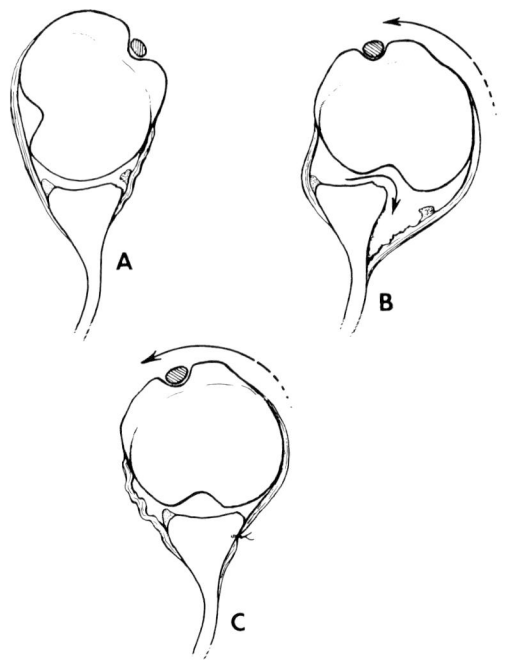

FIGURE 7
A, Mechanics of Hill-Sachs lesion in a patient with a Bankart lesion. (Reproduced with permission from Warner JJP, Caborn DNM: Overview of shoulder instability. *Crit Rev Phys Rehab Med* 1992; 4:145-198.) **B,** With external rotation, the anterior capsule fails to develop tension and the humeral head moves anteriorly as it rotates and dislocates when the Hill-Sachs defect comes in contact with the anterior glenoid rim. **C,** Repair of the Bankart lesion allows the anterior capsule to develop tension with external rotation, so the humeral head remains centered on the glenoid.

of longer duration, recurrent dislocations, and inferior displacement of the humeral head.[102,105] Very rarely, when the Hill-Sachs lesion involves more than 30% of the humeral articular surface, there is concern that it may contribute to anterior instability independent of ligament damage.[19,20] It is believed that external rotation allows the posterior humeral head defect to come in contact with the anterior glenoid rim, thus allowing the humeral head to fall out of the glenoid cavity (Fig. 7). However, surgical procedures that either eliminate the humeral head defect (eg, infraspinatus tendon transfer, humeral head replacement, or allograft reconstruction)[6,20,105] (Christian Gerber, MD, personal communication) or rotate it out of contact with the glenoid by a proximal humeral osteotomy[84,85] are rarely indicated. In the vast majority of cases, the humeral head defect is small and is believed to play only a minor role in the perpetuation of shoulder instability;[19,20] anterior capsular repair is all that is needed to correct the instability. Anterior humeral head defects seen in cases of locked posterior

dislocations have greater importance but are rarely seen in recurrent instability.

LABRUM

Many studies have examined the morphologic variability of the glenoid labrum and its role in instability.[7,106-112] This structure probably contributes to stability of the glenohumeral joint through three mechanisms. First, it acts as a fibrocartilaginous ring around the glenoid to which the capsuloligamentous structures are anchored.[1-3,14,108,111] Second, it deepens the concavity of the glenoid socket to an average of 9 mm and 5 mm in the superior-inferior and anterior-posterior planes, respectively (Fig. 8).[113-115] This acts in a manner analogous to a chock-block that prevents a wheel from

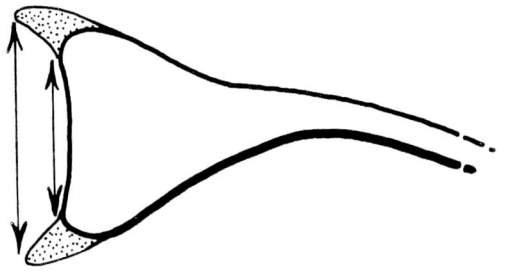

FIGURE 8
The glenoid labrum increases the surface area and depth of the glenoid socket. (Reproduced with permission from Warner JJP, Caborn DNM: Overview of shoulder instability. *Crit Rev Phys Rehab Med* 1992; 4:145-198.)

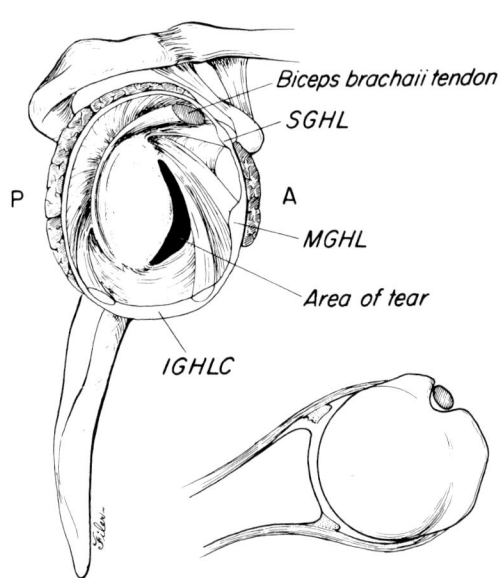

FIGURE 9
Anatomy of the Bankart lesion (see text). (Reproduced with permission from Warner JJP, Caborn DNM: Overview of shoulder instability. *Crit Rev Phys Rehab Med* 1992; 4:145-198.)

rolling down a hill. Loss of the glenoid labrum, as with a Bankart lesion, can decrease the glenoid socket depth by up to 50%.[113] Third, the glenoid labrum can enhance stability of the joint by increasing the surface area of contact for the humeral head.[88,114,115] Thus, it can increase the GH_I by acting as a loadbearing structure (Fig. 8).

The most common pathology affecting the labrum is a Bankart lesion.[1,2,22] Functionally, this lesion represents a detachment of the anchoring point of the inferior glenohumeral ligament (IGHL) and middle glenohumeral ligament (MGHL) on the glenoid rim, decreasing the depth of the glenoid (Fig. 9). This lesion should not be confused with the normal anatomic variants of a sublabral sulcus underneath a cord-like MGHL or a loosely attached labrum superiorly. In general, the labrum is closely attached to the glenoid below its equator; however, above the equator of the glenoid the labrum may be applied only loosely (Fig. 10).[108] Virtually all labral lesions are associated with glenohumeral instability.[110,112,116-118]

NEGATIVE INTRA-ARTICULAR PRESSURE

Kumar and Balasubramianiam[119] demonstrated that venting a cadaver shoulder joint to atmosphere resulted in marked inferior translation when the arm was adducted. They concluded that capsular structures played little role in stability when the arm was in this position. Basmajian and Bazant[68] and others,[27,65-67,75] however, suggested that inferior stability is afforded by tension that develops in the superior and coracohumeral ligaments as the humeral head slides inferiorly on the glenoid surface, which is inclined superiorly.

However, it seems likely that when the arm is hanging at the side, the muscles of the shoulder are often relaxed and the glenoid faces slightly inferiorly, so that neither rotator cuff contraction nor tension in the superior capsular structures resists inferior translation of the humeral head.[42,43,120] In such situations, negative pressure within the joint may play an important role in limiting inferior translation of the humeral head.

The biomechanical explanation for the negative intra-articular pressure (NIP) effect is represented in Figure 11. The glenohumeral joint can be described as a closed compartment surrounded by an elastic diaphragm (joint capsule). If the articular surfaces are pulled apart, a negative pressure or suction effect develops to resist further displacement. The magnitude of this pressure gradient has been shown to be about -42 cm of water in the adducted, relaxed shoulder,[121] perhaps due to high osmotic pressure in the interstitial tissues that causes water to be drawn out of the joint.[122] When a 25 N inferior force was applied to a cadaver shoulder, this pressure gradient dropped to -82 cm water. Any condition that vents the capsule or increases joint volume

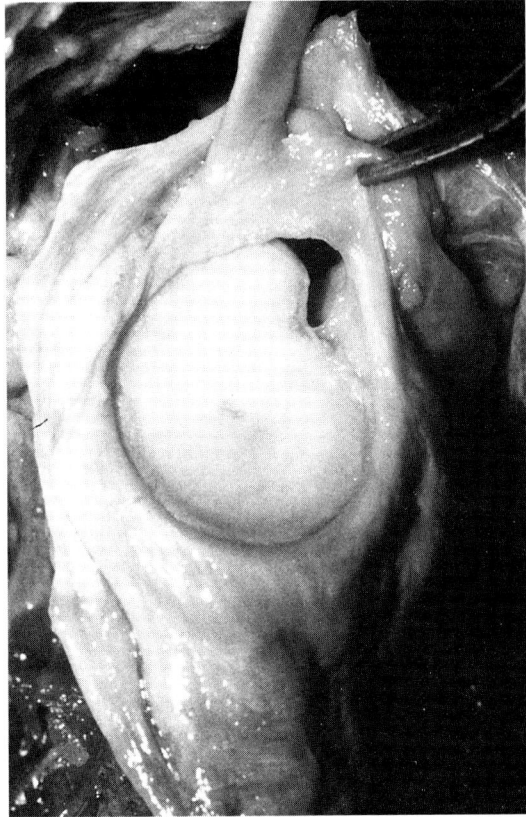

FIGURE 10
Loosely attached glenoid labrum above the equator of the glenoid is a normal anatomic variation. (Reproduced with permission from Cooper DE, Arnoczky SP, O'Brien SJ, et al: Anatomy, histology, and vascularity of the glenoid labrum. *J Bone Joint Surg* 1992;74A:46-52.)

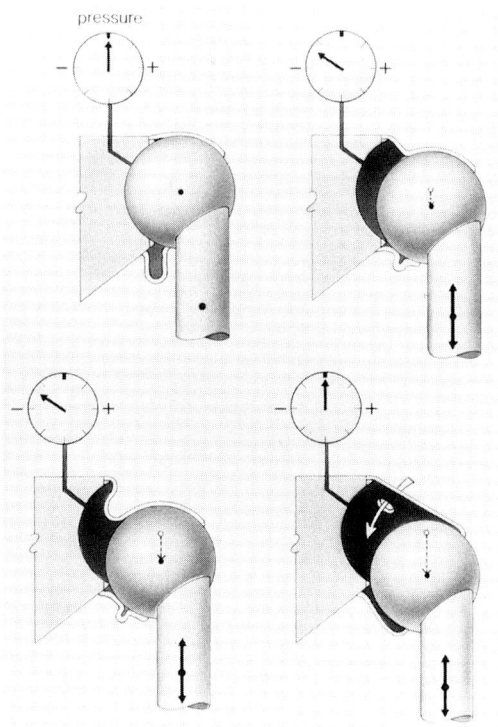

FIGURE 11
The role of negative intra-articular pressure in inferior stability of the glenohumeral joint. **Top left** and **top right,** In the normal, closed joint compartment, the weight of the arm tending to subluxate the humeral head inferiorly on the glenoid is resisted by the negative pressure or vacuum effect created by a sealed capsular space. **Bottom left** and **bottom right,** In a shoulder with a lax capsule or larger joint volume (bottom left), the humeral head may translate further inferiorly before the negative pressure is sufficient to resist additional translation. In a shoulder with a capsular tear or a rotator interval capsular defect, the volume of the joint compartment is vented and the vacuum effect is lost. The humeral head may now move inferiorly until tension in the superior capsule resists inferior translation. (Reproduced with permission from Pagnani MJ, Warren RF: The pathophysiology of anterior shoulder instability. *Sports Med Arthroscopy Rev* 1993;1:177-189.)

will reduce the restraining effect of NIP. For example, a capsular tear or a "rotator interval" defect will vent the capsule and eliminate the vacuum effect of NIP (Fig. 11).

The magnitude of the NIP effect on limitation of joint motion depends on arm position and muscle activity.[28,48,123,124] Warner and associates[28] showed experimentally that in the adducted cadaver shoulder, venting the capsule resulted in a wide range of inferior translation (2 to 20 mm) when a 50 N inferior force was applied to the humerus. However, when the shoulder was passively abducted, venting the capsule increased inferior translation only a few millimeters. This is due to tension in the IGHL complex when the arm is abducted.

CAPSULOLIGAMENTOUS STRUCTURES
The shoulder joint capsule is composed of a variably thick layer of tissue, with discrete thickenings that constitute glenohumeral ligaments (Fig. 12).[7,31,32] Most knowledge of this anatomy has come from cadaver dissections[7,30,125-129] or observations during surgery.[3,8,11-14,17,19,22,23,130-132] DePalma and associates[7] noted the variability of

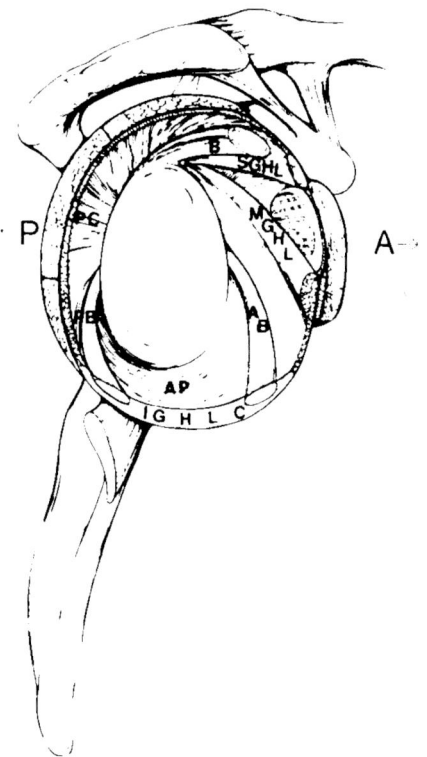

FIGURE 12
Capsuloligamentous anatomy, viewed from the side with the anterior aspect (A) to the right and the posterior aspect (P) to the left. The humeral head has been removed, leaving the glenoid. The superior (SGHL) and middle (MGHL) ligaments are labelled. The inferior glenohumeral ligament (IGHL) complex consists of an anterior band (AB), posterior band (PB), and the interposed axillary pouch (AP). The posterior capsule (PC) is the area above the posterior band (PB). The biceps (B) is also labelled. (Reproduced with permission from O'Brien SJ, et al: The anatomy and histology of the inferior glenohumeral ligament complex of the shoulder. *Am J Sports Med* 1990;18:449-456.)

this capsuloligamentous apparatus and described six types of anatomic arrangements based on the pattern of synovial recesses. They believed that these patterns might correlate with the risk for shoulder instability. With the advent of arthroscopy, the marked variability in size and appearance of the glenohumeral ligaments has been confirmed.[27,29,45] Furthermore, the amount of passive translation of the humeral head on the glenoid correlates with both arm position and size of these ligaments.[26,27] These observations confirmed the impressions of Turkel and associates[133] that different portions of the capsuloliga-

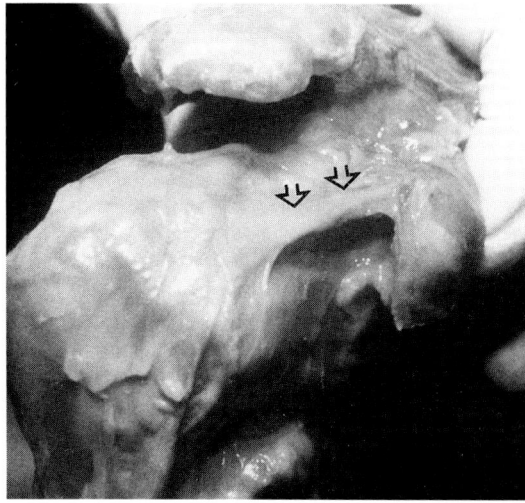

FIGURE 13
Coaracohumeral ligament anatomy (arrows) (see text).

mentous complex provide static stability, depending on arm position and the direction of an applied load tending to displace the humeral head out of the glenoid. Most recent work has attempted to clarify the static role of each portion of the glenohumeral joint capsule. These studies have consisted of radiographic measurements,[29,133] strain gauge analysis,[134,135] selective ligament cutting experiments,[27,44,45,124,136-142] and material property analysis.[51-53,63,143]

The anatomy and role of each of the glenohumeral ligaments are briefly described below.

Superior and Coracohumeral Ligament Although there is some controversy concerning the relative importance of the superior glenohumeral ligament (SGHL) and the coracohumeral ligament (CHL), they are described together because their anatomic courses are parallel. The ligaments constitute the structural components of the "rotator interval" region.[15,22,32,44,131,132,144,145] This is a triangular-shaped space between the anterior border of the supraspinatus tendon and the upper border of the subscapularis tendon. The CHL is an extra-articular structure that originates on the lateral surface of the coracoid process and fans out to insert into the greater and lesser tuberosities of the proximal humerus on either side of the bicipital groove (Fig. 13). This is thought to be the major structural component of the anterior-superior capsule;[15,37,68,124,131,132,146] however, Cooper and associates[147] showed histologic evidence that the CHL is a capsular fold rather than a true ligament. Others have found the CHL to be a thick, cord-like ligamentous structure with about four times the cross-sectional area and strength of the SGHL.[145]

The SGHL originates from the superior glenoid rim, just inferior to the biceps tendon, runs parallel to the CHL, and inserts into the lesser tuberosity of the humerus just medial to the bicipital groove. Although quite variable in size, it is the most consistent glenohumeral ligament, because it is demonstrable in more than 90% of cases.[7,27,29,31,32,45,147] The CHL, rather than the SGHL, possesses the stiffness and loadbearing capacity to statically stabilize the humeral head in the glenoid; however, the stiffness of the CHL is only 15% of the value reported for the anterior cruciate ligament (ACL) of the knee.[146]

The current consensus from experimental and clinical observations is that these two structures constrain the humeral head on the glenoid, limiting inferior translation and external rotation when the arm is adducted and posterior translation when the shoulder is in a position of forward flexion, adduction, and internal rotation (Fig. 14).[142]

Middle Glenohumeral Ligament The MGHL is the most variable of the glenohumeral ligaments, being absent in up to 30% of cases and poorly defined in another 10%.[7,27,29,31,32,45] It originates from the superior glenoid just below the SGHL and above the anterior band of the IGHL, slightly medial to the glenoid labrum. It has two morphologic variations: sheetlike and confluent with the anterior band of the IGHL or cordlike with a foraminal separation between it and the anterior band of the IGHL.

Experimental studies and clinical observations have suggested that the MGHL functions to statically limit anterior translation of the humeral head when the arm is abducted in the range from 60° to 90°, in external rotation, and during inferior translation when the arm is adducted at the side (Fig. 14).[27,29,133,134]

Inferior Glenohumeral Ligament Complex The IGHL complex has been described as a triangular-shaped structure that runs from the labrum to the humeral head between the subscapularis and triceps.[7] It has a thickened anterior edge, called the superior band.[133] Histologic studies suggest that this structure is a three-component complex composed of discrete anterior bands (ABs) and posterior bands (PBs) with an interposed axillary pouch (Fig. 12);[31] however, Ticker and associates[148] have found the posterior band to be an inconsistent structure. Performing precise thickness measurements, they found the superior band to be the thickest region, and found all regions of the IGHL complex to be thicker near the glenoid than the

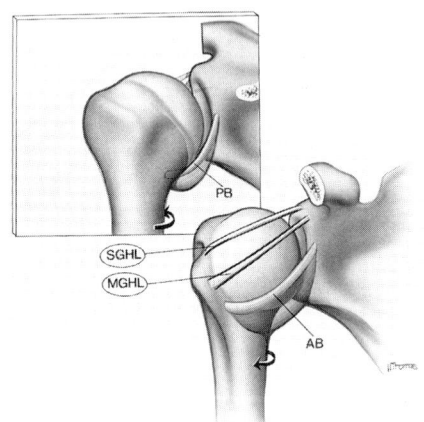 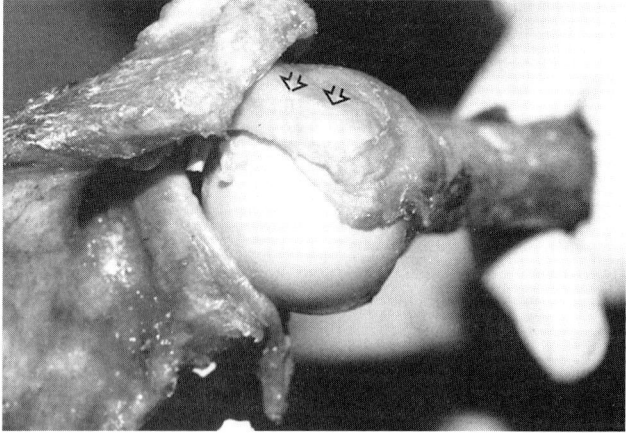

FIGURE 14
Left, The superior (SGHL) and middle (MGHL) glenohumeral ligaments are taut in adduction and external rotation. The anterior (AB) and posterior (PB) bands of the inferior glenohumeral ligament complex are lax in this position. (Reproduced with permission from Warner JJP, Deng X, et al: Static capsuloligamentous restraints to superior-inferior translation of the glenohumeral joint. *Am J Sports Med* 1992;20:675-685.) **Right,** Role of the coracohumeral and superior glenohumeral ligaments (arrows) in posterior stability when the shoulder is positioned in forward flexion, adduction, and internal rotation.

humerus.[148] With abduction, this complex moves underneath the humeral head, becoming taut in the fashion of a hammock (Fig. 15). Depending on rotation of the humeral head, the entire complex functions to constrain anterior, posterior, and inferior translations of the abducted shoulder. Internal rotation causes the entire hammock-like complex to move posterior to the humeral head, thus limiting posterior translation; external rotation causes the entire IGHL complex to move anteriorly, thus statically limiting anterior translation (Fig. 15).[27,31] Horizontal flexion of the abducted shoulder tightens the posterior portion of the IGHL complex so that both posterior and anterior translation are limited, while horizontal extension tightens the anterior portion, thus limiting anteroposterior translation.[45] Although the IGHL complex statically limits inferior translation of the abducted shoulder joint, it has only a secondary role in adduction because it forms a dependent fold (Figs. 14 and 15).[27]

Posterior Capsule (PC) This region of the capsule is posterior and superior to the posterior band of the IGHL complex.[31,32] There is little anatomic information available on this region of the capsule, although many surgeons and anatomists have commented that it is the thinnest portion of the joint capsule.[142,149] Warren and associates[142] and others[136,137] have suggested that it functions as the primary static stabilizer to posterior translation of the adducted, forward flexed, and internally rotated shoulder.

Material Properties of the Joint Capsule Much of our initial understanding of shoulder ligaments was limited to that derived from descriptive anatomy and surgical observations. Some distortion is inevitably introduced, however. For example, arthroscopic inspection of ligamentous and capsular structures examines only the surface synovial side of the capsule. Thin, flimsy synovial tissue can appear robust and impressive if pleat-

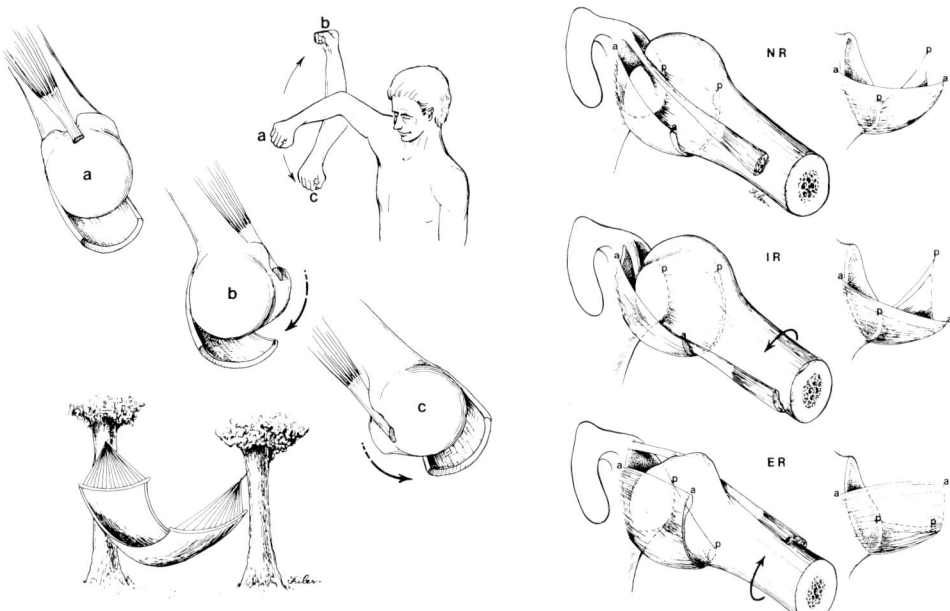

FIGURE 15

Left, The "hammock"-like anatomy of the inferior glenohumeral ligament complex allows for reciprocal tightening of its anterior and posterior portions when the arm moves from neutral rotation in abduction (a) to external (b) and internal (c) rotation. (Reproduced with permission from Warner JJP, Caborn DNM: Overview of shoulder instability. *Crit Rev Phys Rehab Med* 1992; 4:145-198.) **Right,** Orientation changes of the anterior band (aa) and the posterior band (bb) during internal (IR), external (ER), and neutral (NR) rotation. (Reproduced with permission from Warner JJP, Caborn DNM, Berger R, et al: Dynamic capsuloligamentous anatomy of the glenohumeral joint. *J Shoulder Elbow Surg* 1993;2:115-133.)

ed or folded by arm rotation. Conversely, a significant capsular thickening may be indistinguishable from the surrounding capsule. Until recently, few studies examined the precise structure, composition, and material properties of the IGHL complex.

The maximum tensile strength of the anterior-inferior capsule averages 70 N (approximately 20 kg). This value decreases after age 50.[63,143] Bigliani and associates[51] measured the dimensions of the IGHL complex and analyzed its strength and failure modes using tensile testing. They showed that the superior portion (anterior band region) had the greatest thickness, averaging 2.8 mm, while the posterior region was the thinnest, with an average thickness of 1.70 mm. Stress at failure was similar for the three regions of the IGHL complex, averaging 5.5 Mpa, far lower than that of knee ligaments. Thus, in the shoulder, the ligaments must share load with the muscles and other stabilizing mechanisms. The predominant modes of failure are at the glenoid insertion (analogous to a Bankart lesion) and in the midsubstance (as might be expected in capsular stretching and laxity). However, there is significant midsubstance ligament strain prior to failure, even in specimens that ultimately fail at the glenoid insertion. This suggests that plastic deformation of the capsule may result from submaximal repetitive trauma or a single event. In the latter case, although a Bankart lesion is often the result, stretching of the IGHL complex is a likely concomitant lesion. These concepts are clinically relevant because they support the technical approach of some capsular shift or tensioning at the time of Bankart repair.

Tensile studies on the IGHL complex at faster, more clinically relevant strain rates showed a viscoelastic response in the anterior axillary pouch and superior band regions, both of which became stronger and stiffer at the higher strain rates.[148] These findings suggest a functional adaptability of different regions of the IGHL complex to restrain the humeral head at various loading rates.

Ticker and associates[150] compared dumbbell-shaped specimens cut from the IGHL complex with bone-ligament-bone preparations tested in tension and studied the regions of the IGHL complex biomechanically and histologically. The results of these studies suggested that the central portion of the ligament has a more elastic behav-ior, while the insertion areas near the humerus and glenoid are more viscoelastic and have a less oriented collagen organization and a higher proteoglycan content.

Thus, the IGHL complex would appear to be a complex structure capable of adjusting to high-speed athletic loading as well as to prolonged, low-level use. Much remains to be elucidated about this important structure. For example, the effect of repetitive fatigue loading is largely unknown, yet this may be an extremely important mechanism of injury in athletes who subject their shoulders to repetitive minor injuries, usually in different arm positions so that many different areas of the capsule are stressed.

PATHOANATOMY OF THE CAPSULOLIGAMENTOUS STRUCTURES

Bankart Lesion A Bankart lesion occurs when the anterior portion of the IGHL complex detaches from its glenoid attachment after fracture or soft-tissue rupture (Fig. 9).[1,2,22] Although this lesion has been shown experimentally[58] and clinically[26] to increase anterior translation of the humeral head on the glenoid when an anterior drawer is applied, complete dislocation requires associated capsular injury.[1,2,6,8,17,22,51,58] Indeed, the translations that result from just an isolated Bankart lesion are quite small.[58] This may account for the higher failure rate seen after arthroscopic Bankart repair, because these "minimally invasive" procedures do not cause scarring of the lax capsule, while open approaches, even those that purport only to repair the Bankart lesion, may reduce elasticity of the IGHL complex due to scarring from the open approach.

Capsular Injury Capsular rupture or stretching is a recognized consequence in many cases of traumatic anterior shoulder dislocation.[14,19,20,22,25,151,152] Reeves[61,62] showed capsular rupture in 55% of the anterior dislocations treated and Symeonides[24] believed that 15% in a series of anterior dislocations had both labral detachment and anterior capsular ruptures. Neer[131,132] and Altchek and associates[59] described patients with traumatic anterior-inferior instability who had concomitant capsular laxity or injury along with a Bankart lesion. More recently, Johnson[152] reported that 54% of 121 shoulders that underwent arthroscopy acutely after an anterior dislocation had disruption of the glenohumeral ligaments. This concept of combined Bankart lesion and capsular laxity has treatment implications because an anatomic surgical reconstruction would correct these two components of capsuloligamentous injury to the extent that they are present.

CAPSULAR LAXITY

Laxity of the glenohumeral joint capsule is a requirement of normal glenohumeral rotation. Experimental and clinical studies have shown that the degree of this laxity varies among individuals.[27,28,33-35,37,44] It is unclear whether excessive (constitutional) laxity is a risk factor for clinical instability of the shoulder joint. Emery and Mullaji[36] found that more than 75% of preadolescents had shoulder joints that could be asymptomatically subluxated on examination. O'Driscoll and Evans[50] and Warner and associates[26] found that individuals undergoing surgery for anterior instability often had a contralateral, "normal" shoulder that could be subluxated or dislocated under anesthesia. Uthoff and Piscopo[49] also suggested that constitutional hyperlaxity of the glenohumeral joint may predispose to clinical instability.

Laxity is assessed as passive movement of the humeral head relative to the glenoid when the shoulder girdle muscles are relaxed or paralyzed by anesthesia. There is a clinical debate as to the usefulness of laxity assessment by drawer testing under anesthesia.[26,27,33-35,37,44,46,47,59] Certainly there is an overlap between normal laxity and clinical instability. Nevertheless, the technique of drawer testing under anesthesia can be useful if one bears in mind the effect of arm position on tension in different portions of the capsule. For example, a large sulcus sign with the arm adducted at the side is correlated with laxity of the SGHL and CHL as well as the IGHL complex. If this sulcus sign persists during external rotation of the adducted shoulder, it is likely that there will be marked laxity or deficiency of the SGHL, CHL, and MGHL (Fig. 16).[27,153] Furthermore, although anterior translation of the humeral head on the glenoid may be over 1 cm when a drawer test is performed on a normal shoulder,[45] this should reduce to only a few millimeters when the arm is abducted and externally rotated. If the humeral head can be subluxated over the glenoid in this position, there is significant laxity or injury to the IGHL complex.

PROPRIOCEPTION

Specialized nerve endings, proprioceptive mechanoreceptors (Pacinian corpuscles, Ruffini endings, Golgi tendon-like endings), have been described in the capsule and ligaments of the glenohumeral joint.[154,155] These neuroreceptors transduce electric signals that give information about joint position and motion.[156,157] Lephart and associates[38] and Blasier and associates[39] have postulated that stimulation of these capsuloligamentous mechanoreceptors in the shoulder joint by pressure or tension in the ligaments during joint rotation results in a reflexive contraction of the muscles about the joint, thus controlling sudden accelerations and decelerations of the humerus in the glenoid. Therefore, the capsule and ligaments of the shoulder may not only act to statically control motion of the joint, but can

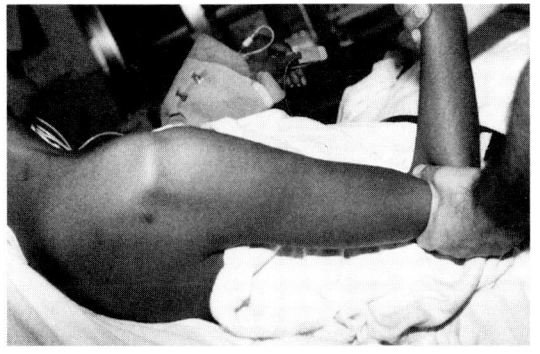 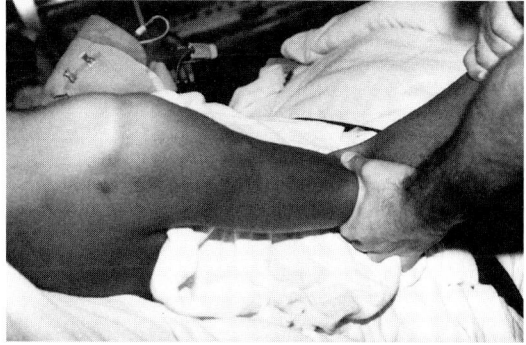

FIGURE 16
A large sulcus sign in neutral rotation (**left**) that persists in external rotation (**right**) suggests laxity of the superior capsular structures.

also provide afferent feedback for reflexive muscular control of the rotator cuff and biceps tendon. This kind of mechanism probably helps protect the joint against excessive translations and rotations that might otherwise lead to soft-tissue injury and instability.[38-40] Lephart and associates[38] have shown that there is a significant deficit of normal proprioception in an unstable shoulder and that surgical repair restores normal proprioception.

DYNAMIC FACTORS

Dynamic stability of the glenohumeral joint is achieved through active contraction of the rotator cuff and long head of the biceps brachi. Stability is achieved through three mechanisms: (1) joint compression of matching concave-convex surfaces; (2) synergistic, coordinated contraction of the rotator cuff muscles, acting to steer the humeral head into the glenoid in different positions of arm rotation; and (3) dynamization of the glenohumeral ligaments through direct attachments of rotator cuff tendons. A coordinated scapulothoracic rhythm is also required to provide a stable glenoid platform for the humeral head during arm rotation.

Normal rotator cuff activity is also necessary to avoid injury to the capsuloligamentous structures. Morrey and Chao[158] calculated that the anterior shear force in the abducted and externally rotated shoulder is about 60 kg. The tendency for anterior displacement of the humeral head must be resisted by both static restraints (capsule and ligaments) and dynamic restraints (rotator cuff and long head of the biceps). Furthermore, contraction of the rotator cuff and biceps when the arm is in this position significantly reduces strain in the anterior capsule.[159-164] Because the maximum tensile strength of the anterior capsule averages about 20 kg under extreme loading conditions, such as a fall with the arm in an abducted and externally rotated position, the capsule would fail if not for the protective effect of rotator cuff contraction. As previously suggested, proprioceptive feedback from capsular stretch may mediate this reflexive contraction of the rotator cuff.[38-40] Another example of the importance of rotator cuff contraction is the patient who has a seizure that results in a posterior dislocation from asynchronous contraction of the internal rotators.

Patients older than 50 years have an increased incidence of rotator cuff tear with anterior shoulder dislocation. This has been termed the "posterior mechanism" of shoulder dislocation and appears to be caused by greater age-related attrition in the cuff tendons than in the anterior capsule.[63,165] Furthermore, subscapularis tendon rupture may also occur with shoulder dislocation in older individuals.[9,11-13,18,54,65,166-168]

JOINT COMPRESSION EFFECT
Compression of the articular surface provided by contraction of the rotator cuff and long head of the biceps brachi enhances joint stability by increasing the conforming fit of the humeral head into the glenoid. Howell and Galinat[113] described this effect as the "containment concept" and suggested that it was a more important stabilizing mechanism than a coordinated and balanced functioning rotator cuff.[169] Lippitt and associates[115] described this effect as "concavity compression" and demonstrated that if the glenoid depth was decreased by removing a portion of the labrum, the stability of the joint was markedly reduced. Bowen and associates[114] used ligament cutting studies to show that joint compression was much more important to inferior stability than static capsular constraints. Blasier and associates[170] quantified the efficiencies of the dynamic stabilizers.

The clinical consequence of weak or ineffective rotator cuff action is that it allows greater degrees of translation of the humeral head on the glenoid during active shoulder motion. This can sometimes be seen in an overhead athlete with a "lax" shoulder joint who develops pain. Arthroscopy may show partial injury to the rotator cuff along with fraying or injury to the labrum. Rotator cuff strengthening programs can provide additional stability by improving muscle tone and coordination during repetitive overhead motions.[171]

COORDINATED ROTATOR CUFF CONTRACTION
Inman and associates[78] and others[42,43,120] have studied two-dimensional forces across the glenohumeral joint by planar vector analysis. More recently, Bassett and associates[172] evaluated three-dimensional orientation of the muscles across the abducted glenohumeral joint. All of these studies have demonstrated the complex

and interdependent role of the rotator cuff muscles in controlling shoulder motion and stability.

Jobe and associates and others have demonstrated normal and abnormal patterns of muscle activity in individuals with and without shoulder instability, respectively.[173-178] Furthermore, Warner and associates[37] demonstrated that patients with shoulder instability had altered rotator cuff strength patterns compared to normal controls. The posterior rotator cuff and biceps tendon reduce strain in the IGHL and also reduce anterior translation in the abducted externally rotated shoulder.[159-163,179] Therefore, it is possible to understand how fatigue in the rotator cuff muscles of a throwing athlete might place the anterior capsuloligamentous structures at risk for injury during repetitive overhead motions.[40] An additional clinical example of the importance of rotator cuff contraction in stability of the joint is provided by patients with voluntary instability who can cause dislocation by asynchronous contraction of the muscles about the shoulder.[180]

LIGAMENT DYNAMIZATION

The glenohumeral ligaments and capsule are relatively lax in the midranges of shoulder rotation and function only at the end ranges to limit excessive translation and rotation of the humeral head on the glenoid.[27,29,33-35,44,133] Clarke and associates[181] and Ferrari[30] have demonstrated that the rotator cuff tendons attach directly to portions of the capsuloligamentous apparatus. Therefore, it is possible that during active shoulder motion the capsule and ligaments may be "dynamized," or placed under tension by contraction of the tendons of the rotator cuff. Although the orientation and length changes of these ligaments have been documented by recent anatomic studies,[29] the direct effect of

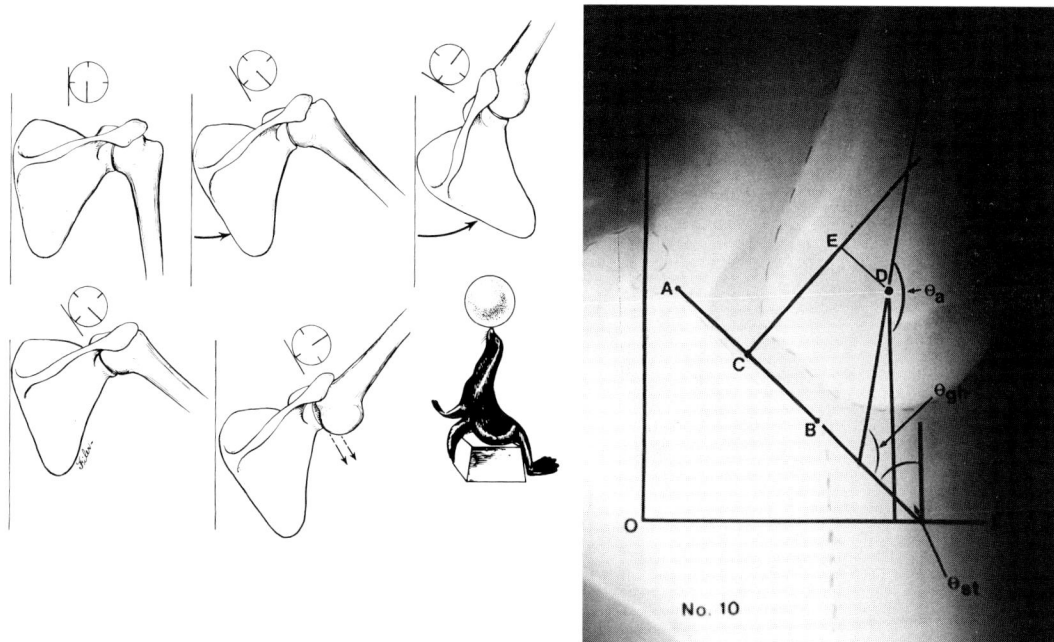

FIGURE 17
Top left, Normal scapulothoracic rotation positions the glenoid underneath the humeral head so that it acts as a stable platform. **Bottom left,** Failure of proper scapulothoracic motion results in loss of the stable glenoid platform underneath the humeral head. This is analogous to a seal balancing a ball on its nose. (Reproduced with permission from Warner JJP, Caborn DNM: Overview of shoulder instability. *Crit Rev Phys Rehab Med* 1992; 4:145-198.) **Right,** Radiographic measurements in a patient with inferior subluxation of the humeral head due to failure of proper scapulothoracic rotation in abduction. Glenohumeral rotation (gh) is much greater than scapulothoracic rotation (st), therefore, at maximum abduction of the arm (a) the glenoid is not in a stable position underneath the humeral head. The center of the glenoid is marked by a line (CE) bisecting a line (AB) tangent to the glenoid surface. The center of the humeral head (D) is inferior to this.

rotator cuff contraction on the capsule and ligaments remains to be clarified.

KINEMATICS: EFFECT OF SCAPULOTHORACIC MOTION

The glenohumeral and scapulothoracic joints must function in a normal, coordinated, and intercalated manner if glenohumeral motion and stability are to be normal.[5,27,28,66-68,75,182] Although there may be some individual variations, the normal scapulohumeral rhythm motion relationship is 2° of glenohumeral rotation for every 1° of scapulothoracic rotation during scapular plane abduction.[42,43] Both clinical and radiographic studies have documented that patients with shoulder instability can have abnormal scapulothoracic motion.[41,182,183] Furthermore, electromyographic (EMG) studies have demonstrated that fatigue of the serratus anterior and trapezius may occur with repetitive overhead activities and may lead to poor scapulothoracic control.[173,178,184]

Whether this scapulothoracic dysfunction is a primary or a secondary phenomenon with respect to instability, it has several biomechanical consequences for glenohumeral joint motion. First, if the scapula does not properly rotate during glenohumeral rotation, the glenoid will not be in a position to act as a stable platform on which the humeral head can rotate, which might increase strain in the glenohumeral ligaments and ultimately contribute to instability (Fig. 17). Second, if the scapula wings, the coracoacromial arch will descend relative to the advancing greater tuberosity of a flexing glenohumeral joint, which could result in "nonoutlet impingement."[41] Furthermore, we have seen several cases of individuals who were treated for primary shoulder instability when they had a long thoracic nerve injury that resulted in scapular winging and secondary instability. These observations support the need to carefully assess scapulothoracic function in all patients with suspected instability and also to include axioscapular muscle strengthening in any rehabilitation program for shoulder instability.

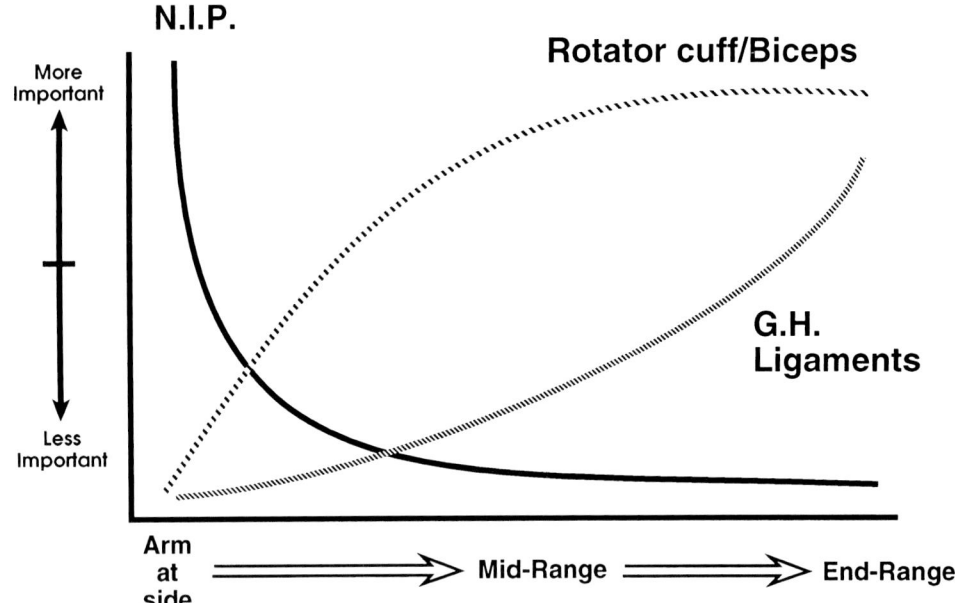

GLENOHUMERAL ROTATION

FIGURE 18
Relative importance of the dynamic and static factors for shoulder stability (see text).

CONCLUSION

Successful clinical management of shoulder instability requires a thorough understanding of all the interdependent static and dynamic factors that maintain normal glenohumeral motion and stability. The relative importance of many of these factors is schematically represented in Figure 18. In addition, all potential pathologic conditions must be considered and carefully ruled out when evaluating any patient with shoulder instability. Because different structural lesions may occur in combination (ie, Bankart lesion, capsular injury, articular injury), all surgery should be directed at anatomic restoration of each of these lesions.

REFERENCES

1. Bankart ASB: The pathology and treatment of recurrent dislocation of the shoulder-joint. *Br J Surg* 1938;26:23-29.

2. Bankart ASB: Recurrent or habitual dislocation of the shoulder-joint. *Br Med J* 1923;2:1132-1133.

3. Bost FC, Inman VT: The pathological changes in recurrent dislocation of the shoulder: Report of Bankart's operative procedure. *J Bone Joint Surg* 1942;24:595-613.

4. Caird FM: The shoulder joint in relation to certain dislocations and fractures. *Edinb Med J* 1887;32:708-714.

5. Codman EA (ed): *The Shoulder: Rupture of the Supraspinatus Tendon and Other Lesions in or About the Subacromial Bursa.* Boston, MA, Thomas Todd, 1934.

6. Connolly JF: Humeral head defects associated with shoulder dislocations: Their diagnostic and surgical significance, in American Academy of Orthopaedic Surgeons *Instructional Course Lectures XXI.* St. Louis, MO, CV Mosby, 1972, pp 42-54.

7. DePalma AF, Callery G, Bennett GA: Shoulder joint: Part 1. Variational anatomy and degenerative lesions of the shoulder bone, in Blount WP, Banks SW (eds): American Academy of Orthopaedic Surgeons *Instructional Course Lectures XVI.* Ann Arbor, MI, JW Edwards. 1949, pp 255-281.

8. Flower WH: On pathological changes produced with shoulder joint traumatic dislocation. *Trans Path Soc Lond* 1861;12:179-200.

9. Hawkins RJ, Koppert G: The natural history following anterior dislocation of the shoulder in the older patient. *J Bone Joint Surg* 1982;64B:255.

10. Henry JH, Genung JA: Natural history of glenohumeral dislocation: Revisited. *Am J Sports Med* 1982;10:135-137.

11. McLaughlin HL: Dislocation of the shoulder with tuberosity fracture. *Surg Clin North Am* 1963;43:1615-1620.

12. McLaughlin HL, Cavallaro WU: Primary anterior dislocation of the shoulder. *Am J Surg* 1950;80:615-621.

13. McLaughlin HL, MacLellan DI: Recurrent anterior dislocation of the shoulder: II. A comparative study. *J Trauma* 1967;7:191-201.

14. Moseley HF, Övergaard B: The anterior capsular mechanism in recurrent anterior dislocation of the shoulder: Morphological and clinical studies with special reference to the glenoid labrum and the gleno-humeral ligaments. *J Bone Joint Surg* 1962;44B:913-927.

15. Nobuhara K, Ikeda H: Rotator interval lesion. *Clin Orthop* 1987;223:44-50.

16. Perthes G: Über operationen bei: Habitueller Schulterluxation. *Deutsch Ztschr Chir* 1906;85:199-227.

17. Broca A, Hartmann H: Contribution a L'etude des luxations de l'epaule. *Bull et Memoirs Soc Anat Paris* 1890;4:312-336;416-423.

18. Pettersson G: Rupture of the tendon aponeurosis of the shoulder joint in antero-inferior dislocation: A study on the origin and occurrence of the ruptures. *Acta Chir Scand* 1942;77(suppl):1-187.

19. Rowe CR, Sakellarides HT: Factors related to recurrences of anterior dislocations of the shoulder. *Clin Orthop* 1961;20:40-48.

20. Rowe CR, Zarins B, Ciullo JV: Recurrent anterior dislocation of the shoulder after surgical repair: Apparent causes of failure and treatment. *J Bone Joint Surg* 1984;66A:159-168.

21. Rowe CR: Prognosis in dislocation of the shoulder. *J Bone Joint Surg* 1956;38A:957-977.

22. Rowe CR, Patel D, Southmayd WW: The Bankart procedure: A long-term end-result study. *J Bone Joint Surg* 1978;60A:1-16.

23. Rowe CR, Zarins B: Recurrent transient subluxation of the shoulder. *J Bone Joint Surg* 1981;63A:863-872.

24. Symeonides PP: The significance of the subscapularis muscle in the pathogenesis of recurrent anterior dislocation of the shoulder. *J Bone Joint Surg* 1972;54B:476-483.

25. Townley CO: The capsular mechanism in recurrent dislocation of the shoulder. *J Bone Joint Surg* 1950;32A:370-380.

26. Warner JJP, Janetta-Alpers C, Miller MD: Correlation of glenohumeral laxity with arthroscopic ligament anatomy. *J Shoulder Elbow Surg* 1994;3(suppl):S32.

27. Warner JJ, Deng XH, Warren RF, et al: Static capsuloligamentous restraints to superior-inferior translation of the glenohumeral joint. *Am J Sports Med* 1992;20:675-685.

28. Warner JJP, Deng X, Warren RF, et al: Superoinferior translation in the intact and vented glenohumeral joint. *J Shoulder Elbow Surg* 1993;2:99-105.

29. Warner JJP, Caborn DNM, Berger R, et al: Dynamic capsuloligamentous anatomy of the glenohumeral joint. *J Shoulder Elbow Surg* 1993;2:115-133.

30. Ferrari DA: Capsular ligaments of the shoulder: Anatomical and functional study of the anterior-superior capsule. *Am J Sports Med* 1990;18:20-24.

31. O'Brien SJ, Neves MC, Arnoczky SP, et al: The anatomy and histology of the inferior glenohumeral ligament complex of the shoulder. *Am J Sports Med* 1990;18:449-456.

32. O'Brien SJ, Arnoczky SP, Warren RF, et al: Developmental anatomy of the shoulder and anatomy of the glenohumeral joint, in Rockwood CA Jr, Matsen FA III (eds): *The Shoulder.* Philadelphia, PA, WB Saunders, 1990, vol 1, pp 1-33.

33. Harryman DT II, Sidles JA, Clark JM, et al: Translation of the humeral head on the glenoid with passive glenohumeral motion. *J Bone Joint Surg* 1990;72A:1334-1343.

34. Harryman DT II, Sidles JA, Harris SL, et al: Laxity of the normal glenohumeral joint: A quantitative in vivo assessment. *J Shoulder Elbow Surg* 1992;1:66-76.

35. Lippitt SB, Harris SL, Harryman DT II, et al: In vivo quantification of the laxity of normal and unstable glenohumeral joints. *J Shoulder Elbow Surg* 1994;3:215-223.

36. Emery RJ, Mullaji AB: Glenohumeral joint instability in normal adolescents: Incidence and significance. *J Bone Joint Surg* 1991;73B:406-408.

37. Warner JJ, Micheli LJ, Arslanian LE, et al: Patterns of flexibility, laxity, and strength in normal shoulders and shoulders with instability and impingement. *Am J Sports Med* 1990;18:366-375.

38. Lephart SM, Warner JJP, Borsa PA, et al: Proprioception of the shoulder joint in healthy, unstable, and surgically repaired shoulders. *J Shoulder Elbow Surg* 1994;3:371-380.

39. Blasier RB, Carpenter JE, Huston LJ: Shoulder proprioception: Effect of joint laxity, joint position, and direction of motion. *Orthop Rev* 1994;23:45-50.

40. Carpenter JE, Blasier RB, Pellizzon GG: The effect of muscular fatigue on shoulder proprioception. *Trans Orthop Res Soc* 1993;18:311.

41. Warner JJ, Micheli LJ, Arslanian LE, et al: Scapulothoracic motion in normal shoulders and shoulders with glenohumeral instability and impingement syndrome: A study using Moire topographic analysis. *Clin Orthop* 1992;285:191-199.

42. Poppen NK, Walker PS: Forces at the glenohumeral joint in abduction. *Clin Orthop* 1978;135:165-170.

43. Poppen NK, Walker PS: Normal and abnormal motion of the shoulder. *J Bone Joint Surg* 1976;58A:195-201.

44. Harryman DT II, Sidles JA, Harris SL, et al: The role of the rotator interval capsule in passive motion and stability of the shoulder. *J Bone Joint Surg* 1992;74A:53-66.

45. Schwartz RE, O'Brien SJ, Warren RF, et al: Capsular restraints to anterior-posterior motion of the shoulder: A biomechanical study. *Orthop Trans* 1988;12:727.

46. Cofield RH, Irving JF: Evaluation and classification of shoulder instability: With special reference to examination under anesthesia. *Clin Orthop* 1987;223:32-43.

47. Gerber C, Ganz R: Clinical assessment of instability of the shoulder: With special reference to anterior and posterior drawer tests. *J Bone Joint Surg* 1984;66B:551-556.

48. Helmig P, Sojbjerg JO, Sneppen O, et al: Glenohumeral movement patterns after puncture of the joint capsule: An experimental study. *J Shoulder Elbow Surg* 1993;2:209-215.

49. Uhthoff HK, Piscopo M: Anterior capsular redundancy of the shoulder: Congenital or traumatic? An embryological study. *J Bone Joint Surg* 1985;67B:363-366.

50. O'Driscoll SW, Evans DC: Contralateral shoulder instability following anterior repair: An epidemiological investigation. *J Bone Joint Surg* 1991;73B:941-946.

51. Bigliani LU, Pollock RG, Soslowsky LJ, et al: Tensile properties of the inferior glenohumeral ligament. *J Orthop Res* 1992;10:187-197.

52. Mow VC, Bigliani LU, Flatow EL, et al: Material properties of the inferior glenohumeral ligament and the glenohumeral articular cartilage, in Matsen FA III, Fu FH, Hawkins RJ (eds): *The Shoulder: A Balance of Mobility and Stability.* Rosemont, Ill, American Academy Orthopaedic Surgeons, 1993, pp 29-67.

53. Ticker JB, Flatow EL, Pawluk RJ, et al: The inferior glenohumeral ligament: A correlative biomechanical, biochemical, and histological investigation. *Trans Orthop Res Soc* 1993;18:313.

54. Hawkins RJ, Bell RH, Hawkins RH, et al: Anterior dislocation of the shoulder in the older patient. *Clin Orthop* 1986;206:192-195.

55. Hovelius L: Anterior dislocation of the shoulder in teen-agers and young adults: Five-year prognosis. *J Bone Joint Surg* 1987;69A:393-399.

56. Ehgartner K: Has the duration of cast fixation after shoulder dislocations an influence on the frequency of recurrent dislocation? *Arch Orthop Unfallchir* 1977;89:187-190.

57. Arciero RA, Wheeler JH, Ryan JB, et al: Arthroscopic Bankart repair versus nonoperative treatment for acute, initial anterior shoulder dislocations. *Am J Sports Med* 1994;22:589-594.

58. Speer KP, Deng X, Borrero S, et al: Biomechanical evaluation of a simulated Bankart lesion. *J Bone Joint Surg* 1994;76A: 1819-1826.

59. Altchek DW, Warren RF, Skyhar MJ, et al: T-plasty modification of the Bankart procedure for multidirectional instability of the anterior and inferior types. *J Bone Joint Surg* 1991;73A:105-112.

60. Kinnett JG, Warren RF, Jacobs B: Recurrent dislocation of the shoulder after age fifty. *Clin Orthop* 1980;149:164-168.

61. Reeves B: Acute anterior dislocation of the shoulder: Clinical and experimental studies. *Ann R Coll Surg Engl* 1969;44:255-273.

62. Reeves B: Arthrography in acute dislocation of the shoulder. *J Bone Joint Surg* 1966;48B:182.

63. Reeves B: Experiments on the tensile strength of the anterior capsular structures of the shoulder in man. *J Bone Joint Surg* 1968;50B:858-865.

64. Neviaser RJ, Neviaser TJ, Neviaser JS: Concurrent rupture of the rotator cuff and anterior dislocation of the shoulder in the older patient. *J Bone Joint Surg* 1988;70A:1308-1311.

65. Doos SP, Ray GS, Saha AK: Observation of the tilt of the glenoid cavity of the scapula. *J Anat Soc India* 1966;15:114.

66. Saha AK: Mechanics of elevation of the glenohumeral joint: Its application in rehabilitation of flail shoulder in upper brachial plexus injuries and poliomyelitis and in replacement of the upper humerus by prosthesis. *Acta Orthop Scand* 1973;44:668-678.

67. Saha AK: Dynamic stability of the glenohumeral joint. *Acta Orthop Scand* 1971;42:491-505.

68. Basmajian JV, Bazant FJ: Factors preventing downward dislocation of the adducted shoulder joint: An electromyographic and morphological study. *J Bone Joint Surg* 1959;41A:1182-1186.

69. Bestard EA, Schoene HR, Bestard EH: Glenoplasty in the management of recurrent shoulder dislocation. *Contemp Orthop* 1986;12:47-55.

70. Brewer BJ, Wubben RC, Carrera GF: Excessive retroversion of the glenoid cavity: A cause of non-traumatic posterior instability of the shoulder. *J Bone Joint Surg* 1986;68A:724-731.

71. Hill JA, Tkach L: A study of glenohumeral orientation in patients with anterior recurrent shoulder dislocations using computerized axial tomography. *Orthop Trans* 1985;9:47-48.

72. Hurley JA, Anderson TE, Dear W, et al: Posterior shoulder instability: Surgical versus conservative results with evaluation of glenoid version. *Am J Sports Med* 1992;20:396-400.

73. Galinat BJ, Howell SM, Kraft TA: The glenoid-posterior acromion angle: An accurate method of evaluating glenoid version. *Orthop Trans* 1988;12:727.

74. Scott DJ Jr: Treatment of recurrent posterior dislocations of the shoulder by glenoplasty: Report of three cases. *J Bone Joint Surg* 1967;49A:471-476.

75. Itoi E, Motzkin NE, An K-N, et al: Scapular inclination and inferior instability of the shoulder. *J Shoulder Elbow Surg* 1992;1:131-139.

76. Mallon WJ, Brown HR, Vogler JB III, et al: Radiographic and geometric anatomy of the scapula. *Clin Orthop* 1992;277:142-154.

77. Randelli M, Gambrioli PL: Glenohumeral osteometry by computed tomography in normal and unstable shoulders. *Clin Orthop* 1986;208:151-156.

78. Inman VT, Saunders JB, Abbott LC: Observations on the function of the shoulder joint. *J Bone Joint Surg* 1944;26:1-30.

79. Kronberg M, Brostrom L-A, Soderlund V: Retroversion of the humeral head in the normal shoulder and its relationship to the normal range of motion. *Clin Orthop* 1990;253:113-117.

80. Kronberg M, Brostrom L-A: Humeral head retroversion in patients with unstable humeroscapular joints. *Clin Orthop* 1990;260:207-211.

81. Chaudhuri GK, Sengupta A, Saha AK: Rotation osteotomy of the shaft of the humerus for recurrent dislocation of the shoulder: Anterior and posterior. *Acta Orthop Scand* 1974;45:193-198.

82. Cyprien JM, Vasey HM, Burdet A, et al: Humeral retrotorsion and glenohumeral relationship in the normal shoulder and in recurrent anterior dislocation (scapulometry). *Clin Orthop* 1983;175:8-17.

83. Surin V, Blader S, Markhede G, et al: Rotational osteotomy of the humerus for posterior instability of the shoulder. *J Bone Joint Surg* 1990;72A:181-186.

84. Weber BG, Simpson LA, Hardegger F, et al: Rotational humeral osteotomy for recurrent anterior dislocation of the shoulder associated with a large Hill-Sachs lesion. *J Bone Joint Surg* 1984,66A:1443-1450.

85. Weber BG: Recurrent dislocation of the shoulder: Treatment with subcapital rotation-osteotomy. *Acta Orthop Scand* 1974;45:986-988.

86. Soslowsky LJ, Flatow EL, Bigliani LU, et al: Articular geometry of the glenohumeral joint. *Clin Orthop* 1992;285:181-190.

87. Soslowsky LJ, Flatow EL, Bigliani LU, et al: Quantitation of in situ contact areas at the glenohumeral joint: A biomechanical study. *J Orthop Res* 1992;10:524-534.

88. Bowen MK, Deng XH, Hannafin JA, et al: An analysis of the patterns of glenohumeral joint contact and their relationship to the glenoid "bare area." *Trans Orthop Res Soc* 1992;17:496.

89. Kelkar R, Newton PM, Armengol J, et al: Three-dimensional kinematics of the glenohumeral joint during abduction in the scapular plane. *Trans Orthop Res Soc* 1993;18:136.

90. Howell SM, Galinat BJ, Renzi AJ, et al: Normal and abnormal mechanics of the glenohumeral joint in the horizontal plane. *J Bone Joint Surg* 1988;70A:227-232.

91. Morrey BF, Janes JM: Recurrent anterior dislocation of the shoulder: Long-term follow-up of the Putti-Platt and Bankart procedures. *J Bone Joint Surg* 1976;58A:252-256.

92. Kozlowski K, Colavita N, Morris L, et al: Bilateral glenoid dysplasia: Report of 8 cases. *Austral Radiol* 1985;29:174-177.

93. Kozlowski K, Scougall J: Congenital bilateral glenoid hypoplasia: A report of four cases. *Br J Radiol* 1987;60:705-706.

94. Lintner DM, Sebastianelli WJ, Hanks GA, et al: Glenoid dysplasia: A case report and review of the literature. *Clin Orthop* 1992;283:145-148.

95. McClure JG, Raney RB: Anomalies of the scapula. *Clin Orthop* 1975;110:22-31.

96. Owen R: Bilateral glenoid hypoplasia: Report of five cases. *J Bone Joint Surg* 1953;35B:262-267.

97. Pettersson H: Bilateral dysplasia of the neck of the scapula and associated anomalies. *Acta Radiol Diagn* 1981;22:81-84.

98. Resnick D, Walter RD, Crudale AS: Bilateral dysplasia of the scapular neck. *Am J Roentgenol* 1982;139:387-389.

99. Aston JW Jr, Gregory CF: Dislocation of the shoulder with significant fracture of the glenoid. *J Bone Joint Surg* 1973;55A:1531-1533.

100. Steinmann S, Bigliani LU, McIlveen SJ: Glenoid fractures associated with recurrent anterior dislocation of the shoulder. Proceedings of the American Academy of Orthopaedic Surgeons 57th Annual Meeting, New Orleans, LA. Park Ridge, IL, American Academy of Orthopaedic Surgeons, 1990, p 173.

101. Eve FS: A case of sub-coracoid dislocation of the humerus, with the formation of an indentation on the posterior surface of the head, the joint being unopened. *Med Chir Trans Soc London* 1880;63:317-321.

102. Hermodsson I: Röntgenologische Studdien über die Traumatischen und Habituellen Schultergelenkverrenkungen: Nach vorn und Nach Unten. *Acta Radiol* 1934;20(suppl):1-173.

103. Hill HA, Sachs MD: The grooved defect of the humeral head: A frequently unrecognized complication of dislocations of the shoulder joint. *Radiology* 1940;35:690-700.

104. Pavlov H, Warren RF, Weiss CB Jr, et al: The roentgenographic evaluation of anterior shoulder instability. *Clin Orthop* 1985;194:153-158.

105. Flatow EL, Miller SR, Neer CS II: Chronic anterior dislocation of the shoulder. *J Shoulder Elbow Surg* 1993;2:2-10.

106. Andrews JR, Carson WG Jr, McLeod WD: Glenoid labrum tears related to the long head of the biceps. *Am J Sports Med* 1985;13:337-341.

107. Detrisac DA, Johnson LL (eds): *Arthroscopic Shoulder Anatomy: Pathologic and Surgical Implications*. Thorofare, NJ, Slack Inc, 1986.

108. Cooper DE, Arnoczky SP, O'Brien SJ, et al: Anatomy, histology, and vascularity of the glenoid labrum: An anatomical study. *J Bone Joint Surg* 1992;74A:46-52.

109. Hata Y, Nakatsuchi Y, Saitoh S, et al: Anatomic study of the glenoid labrum. *J Shoulder Elbow Surg* 1992;1:207-214.

110. Pappas AM, Goss TP, Kleinman PK: Symptomatic shoulder instability due to lesions of the glenoid labrum. *Am J Sports Med* 1983;11:279-288.

111. Prodromos CC, Ferry JA, Schiller AL, et al: Histological studies of the glenoid labrum from fetal life to old age. *J Bone Joint Surg* 1990;72A:1344-1348.

112. Kohn D: The clinical relevance of glenoid labrum lesions. *Arthroscopy* 1987;3:223-230.

113. Howell SM, Galinat BJ: The glenoid-labral socket: A constrained articular surface. *Clin Orthop* 1989;243:122-125.

114. Bowen MK, Deng XH, Warner JP, et al: The effect of joint compression on stability of the glenohumeral joint. *Trans Orthop Res Soc* 1992;17:289.

115. Lippitt SB, Vanderhooft JE, Harris SL, et al: Glenohumeral stability from concavity-compression: A quantitative analysis. *J Shoulder Elbow Surg* 1993;2:27-35.

116. Altchek DW, Warren RF, Wickiewicz TL, et al: Arthroscopic labral debridement: A three-year follow-up study. *Am J Sports Med* 1992;20:702-706.

117. Cordasco FA, Steinmann S, Flatow EL, et al: Arthroscopic treatment of glenoid labral tears. *Am J Sports Med* 1993;21:425-431.

118. McKernan DJ, Mutschler TA, Rudert MJ, et al: Significance of a partial and full Bankart lesion: A biomechanical ccomparison. *Trans Orthop Res Soc* 1989;14:231.

119. Kumar VP, Balasubramianiam P: The role of atmospheric pressure in stabilising the shoulder: An experimental study. *J Bone Joint Surg* 1985;67B:719-721.

120. Freedman L, Munro RR: Abduction of the arm in the scapular plane: Scapular and glenohumeral movements. A roentgenographic study. *J Bone Joint Surg* 1966;48A:1503-1510.

121. Browne AO, Hoffmeyer P, An KN, et al: The influence of atmospheric pressure on shoulder stability. *Orthop Trans* 1990;14:259.

122. Matsen FA III, Thomas SC, Rockwood CA Jr: Anterior glenohumeral instability, in Rockwood CA Jr, Matsen FA III (eds): *The Shoulder*. Philadelphia, PA, WB. Saunders, 1990, pp 526-622.

123. Gibb TD, Sidles JA, Harryman DT II, et al: The effect of capsular venting on glenohumeral laxity. *Clin Orthop* 1991;268:120-127.

124. Helmig P, Sojbjerg JO, Kjaersgaard-Andersen P, et al: Distal humeral migration as a component of multidirectional shoulder instability: An anatomical study in autopsy specimens. *Clin Orthop* 1990;252:139-143.

125. Delorme DHD: Die Hemmungsbänder des Schultergelenks und ihre bedeutung für die schulterluxationen. *Arch Klin Chir* 1910;92:79-101.

126. Fick R (ed): *Handbuch der Anatomie und Mechanik der Gelenke: Unter Berücksichtigung der bewegenden Muskeln*. Berlin, Germany, Jena G Fischer, 1904.

127. Flood V: Discovery of a new ligament of the shoulder joint. *Lancet* 1829;1:672-673.

128. Dempster WT: Mechanisms of shoulder movement. *Arch Phys Med Rehabil* 1965;46:49-70.

129. Sarrafian SK: Gross and functional anatomy of the shoulder. *Clin Orthop* 1983;173:11-19.

130. Nicola T: Anterior dislocation of the shoulder: The role of the articular capsule. *J Bone Joint Surg* 1942;24:614-616.

131. Neer CS II: Involuntary inferior and multidirectional instability of the shoulder: Etiology, recognition and treatment, in Stauffer ES (ed): American Academy of Orthopaedic Surgeons *Instructional Course Lectures XXXIV*. St. Louis, MO, CV Mosby, 1985, pp 232-238.

132. Neer CS II, Foster CR: Inferior capsular shift for involuntary inferior and multidirectional instability of the shoulder: A preliminary report. *J Bone Joint Surg* 1980;62A:897-908.

133. Turkel SJ, Panio MW, Marshall JL, et al: Stabilizing mechanisms preventing anterior dislocation of the glenohumeral joint. *J Bone Joint Surg* 1981;63A:1208-1217.

134. O'Connell PW, Nuber GW, Mileski RA, et al: The contribution of the glenohumeral ligaments to anterior stability of the shoulder joint. *Am J Sports Med* 1990;18:579-584.

135. Terry GC, Hammon D, France P, et al: The stabilizing function of passive shoulder restraints. *Am J Sports Med* 1991;19:26-34.

136. Ovesen J, Nielsen S: Anterior and posterior shoulder instability: A cadaver study. *Acta Orthop Scand* 1986;57:324-327.

137. Ovesen J, Nielsen S: Posterior instability of the shoulder: A cadaver study. *Acta Orthop Scand* 1986;57:436-439.

138. Ovesen J, Nielsen S: Experimental distal subluxation in the glenohumeral joint. *Arch Orthop Trauma Surg* 1985;104:78-81.

139. Ovesen J, Sojbjerg JO: Transposition of coracoacromial ligament to humerus in treatment of vertical shoulder joint instability: Clinical applicability of experimental technique. *Arch Orthop Trauma Surg* 1987;106:323-326.

140. Ovesen J, Sojberg JO: Lesions in different types of anterior glenohumeral joint dislocation: An experimental study. *Arch Orthop Trauma Surg* 1986;105:216-218.

141. Motzkin NE, Itoi E, Morrey, BF: Contribution of bulk tissues and deltoid to inferior stability of the shoulder. *Trans Orthop Res Soc* 1992;17:494.

142. Warren RF, Kornblatt IB, Marchand R: Static factors affecting posterior shoulder stability. *Orthop Trans* 1984;8:89.

143. Kaltsas DS: Comparative study of the properties of the shoulder joint capsule with those of other joint capsules. *Clin Orthop* 1983;173:20-26.

144. Neer CS II, Satterlee CC, Dalsey RM, et al: The anatomy and potential effects of contracture of the coracohumeral ligament. *Clin Orthop* 1992;280:182-185.

145. Boardman ND, Debski RE, Taskiran E, et al: Structural and anatomic characteristics of the coracohumeral and superior glenohumeral ligament. *Trans Orthop Res Soc* 1995;20:681.

146. Edelson JG, Taitz C, Grishkan A: The coracohumeral ligament: Anatomy of a substantial but neglected structure. *J Bone Joint Surg* 1991;73B:150-153.

147. Cooper DE, O'Brien SJ, Arnoczky SP, et al: The structure and function of the coracohumeral ligament: An anatomic and microscopic study. J Shoulder Elbow Surg 1993;2:70-77.

148. Ticker JB, Bigliani LU, Soslowsky LJ, et al: Viscoelastic and geometric properties of the inferior glenohumeral ligament. *Orthop Trans* 1992;16:304-305.

149. Fronek J, Warren RF, Bowen M: Posterior subluxation of the glenohumeral joint. *J Bone Joint Surg* 1989;71A:205-216.

150. Ticker JB, Flatow EL, Pawluk RJ, et al: The inferior glenohumeral ligament: A correlative biomechanical, biochemical, and histological investigation. *Orthop Trans* 1993;17:721-722.

151. Bach BR, Warren RF, Fronek J: Disruption of the lateral capsule of the shoulder: A cause of recurrent dislocation. *J Bone Joint Surg* 1988;70B:274-276.

152. Johnson LL: Techniques of anterior glenohumeral ligament repair, in Johnson LL (ed): *Arthroscopic Surgery: Principles and Practice,* ed 3. St. Louis, MO, CV Mosby, 1986, vol 2, pp 1405-1420.

153. Warner JJP, Marks PH: Reconstruction of the antero-superior shoulder capsule with the subscapularis tendon: A case report. *J Shoulder Elbow Surg* 1993;2:260-263.

154. Vangsness CT Jr, Ennis M: Neural anatomy of the human glenoid labrum and shoulder ligaments. Proceedings of the American Academy of Orthopaedic Surgeons 59th Annual Meeting, Washington, DC. Park Ridge, IL, American Academy of Orthopaedic Surgeons, 1992, p 205.

155. Jerosch J, Clahsen H, Grosse-Hackmann A, et al: Effects of proprioceptive fibers in the capsule tissue in stabilizing the glenohumeral joint. *Orthop Trans* 1992;16:773.

156. Grigg P: Response of joint afferent neurons in cat medial articular nerve to active and passive movements of the knee. *Brain Res* 1976;118:482-485.

157. Grigg P, Hoffman AH: Calibrating joint capsule mechanoreceptors as in-vivo soft tissue load cells. *J Biomech* 1989;22:781-785.

158. Morrey BF, Chao EYS: Recurrent anterior dislocation of the shoulder: Clinical and anatomic considerations, in Black J, Dumbleton JH (eds): *Clinical Biomechanics: A Case History Approach*. New York, NY, Churchill Livingstone, 1981, pp 24-46.

159. Blasier RB, Goldberg RE, Tothman ED: Anterior shoulder stability: Contributions of rotator cuff forces and the capsular ligaments in a cadaveric model. *J Shoulder Elbow Surg* 1992;1:140-150.

160. Cain PR, Mutschler TA, Fu FH et al: Anterior stability of the glenohumeral joint: A Dynamic model. *Am J Sports Med* 1987;15:144-148.

161. Itoi E, Motzkin NE, Morrey BF, et al: The stabilizing function of the long head of the biceps with the arm in a hanging position. *J Shoulder Elbow Surg* 1994;3:135-142.

162. Itoi E, Kuechle DK, Newman SR, et al: Stabilising function of the biceps in stable and unstable shoulders. *J Bone Joint Surg* 1993;75B:546-550.

163. Itoi E, Newman SR, Kuechle DK, et al: Dynamic anterior stabilisers of the shoulder with the arm in abduction. *J Bone Joint Surg* 1994;76B:834-836.

164. Rodosky MW, Harner CD, Fu FH: The role of the long head of the biceps muscle and superior glenoid labrum in anterior stability of the shoulder. *Am J Sports Med* 1994;22:121-130.

165. Craig EV: The posterior mechanism of acute anterior shoulder dislocations. *Clin Orthop* 1984;190:212-216.

166. Gerber C, Krushell RJ: Isolated rupture of the tendon of the subscapularis muscle: Clinical features in 16 cases. *J Bone Joint Surg* 1991;73B:389-394.

167. Hauser EDW: Avulsion of the tendon of the subscapularis muscle. *J Bone Joint Surg* 1954;36A:139-141.

168. DePalma AF, Cooke AJ, Prabhakar M: The role of the subscapularis in recurrent anterior dislocations of the shoulder. *Clin Orthop* 1967;54:35-49.

169. Howell SM, Kraft TA: The role of the supraspinatus and infraspinatus muscles in glenohumeral kinematics of anterior shoulder instability. *Clin Orthop* 1991;263:128-134.

170. Blasier RB, Soslowsky LJ, Malicky DM, et al: Anterior glenohumeral stabilization efficiency in a biomechanical model combining ligamentous and muscular constraints. *J Shoulder Elbow Surg* 1994;3(suppl):S23.

171. Burkhead WZ Jr, Rockwood CA Jr: Treatment of instability of the shoulder with an exercise program. *J Bone Joint Surg* 1992;74A:890-896.

172. Bassett RW, Browne AO, Morrey BF, et al: Glenohumeral muscle force and moment mechanics in a position of shoulder instability. *J Biomech* 1990;23:405-415.

173. Glousman R, Jobe F, Tibone J, et al: Dynamic electromyographic analysis of the throwing shoulder with glenohumeral instability. *J Bone Joint Surg* 1988;70A:220-226.

174. Gowan ID, Jobe FW, Tibone JE, et al: A comparative electromyographic analysis of the shoulder during pitching: Professional versus amateur pitchers. *Am J Sports Med* 1987;15: 586-590.

175. Jobe FW, Tibone JE, Perry J, et al: An EMG analysis of the shoulder in throwing and pitching: A preliminary report. *Am J Sports Med* 1983;11:3-5.

176. Kronberg M, Brostrom L-A, Nemeth G: Differences in shoulder muscle activity between patients with generalized joint laxity and normal controls. *Clin Orthop* 1991;269:181-192.

177. Kronberg M, Nemeth G, Brostrom L-A: Muscle activity and coordination in the normal shoulder: An electromyographic study. *Clin Orthop* 1990;257:76-85.

178. Nuber GW, Jobe FW, Perry J, et al: Fine wire electromyography analysis of muscles of the shoulder during swimming. *Am J Sports Med* 1986;14:7-11.

179. Malicky DM, Blasier RB, Guldberg RE, et al: Anterior glenohumeral stabilization efficiency in a biomechanical model combining ligamentous and muscular constraints. *Trans Orthop Res Soc* 1993;18:314.

180. Rowe CR, Pierce DS, Clark JG: Voluntary dislocation of the shoulder: A preliminary report on a clinical, electromyographic, and psychiatric study of twenty-six patients. *J Bone Joint Surg* 1973;55A:445-460.

181. Clark J, Sidles JA, Matsen FA: The relationship of the glenohumeral joint capsule to the rotator cuff. *Clin Orthop* 1990;254:29-34.

182. Ozaki J: Glenohumeral movements of the involuntary inferior and multidirectional instability. *Clin Orthop* 1989;238:107-111.

183. Leffert RD, Gumley G: The relationship between dead arm syndrome and thoracic outlet syndrome. *Clin Orthop* 1987;223:20-31.

184. Bearn JG: An electromyographic study of the trapezius, deltoid, pectoralis major, biceps and triceps muscles, during static loading of the upper limb. *Anat Rec* 1961;140:103-107.

CLASSIFICATION AND EVALUATION

ROGER G. POLLOCK, MD AND EVAN L. FLATOW, MD

Glenohumeral instability encompasses a spectrum of disorders of varying degree, direction, and etiology. Historically, much of the orthopaedic literature has focused on recurrent anterior dislocation, the most common type of glenohumeral instability. Over the past 10 to 20 years, increased attention has been paid to other types of glenohumeral instability. It is now widely recognized that stabilization procedures that may be successful for one type of instability (eg, anterior dislocation) may not be helpful in treating and may even exacerbate other types of instability (eg, multidirectional type). Careful diagnosis and classification of glenohumeral instabilities will afford the best chance of successful treatment of these disorders.

CLASSIFICATION

Glenohumeral instability is classified according to the timing of diagnosis and frequency of the event, the degree, the direction(s), the etiology of the first occurrence, and whether or not the individual can voluntarily produce the instability (Outline 2). Addressing the timing of diagnosis, the instability is either recognized in the acute period (within several hours or days after injury) or the chronic period (longer than several weeks).

With respect to frequency, the event is classified as the first or primary episode or as a recurrent episode. Fortunately, most episodes of dislocation are diagnosed acutely; however, locked dislocations of the posterior type continue to be missed initially, despite the warnings of several published studies.[1,2] Regarding the degree of instability, a dislocation of the glenohumeral joint occurs when there is a complete separation of the articular surfaces, in which the humeral head usually remains locked outside the joint and requires a reduction to restore joint alignment. A subluxa-

OUTLINE 2

CLASSIFICATION OF GLENOHUMERAL INSTABILITY

I. **Timing/Frequency**
   A. Acute
      1. Primary
      2. Recurrent
   B. Chronic

II. **Degree**
   A. Dislocation
   B. Subluxation

III. **Direction**
   A. Anterior
   B. Posterior
   C. Inferior
   D. Bidirectional
      1. Anterior-inferior
      2. Posterior-inferior
   E. Multidirectional

IV. **Etiology**
   A. Traumatic
   B. Atraumatic
   C. Repetitive microtrauma (overuse)

V. **Volition**
   A. Involuntary
   B. Voluntary
      1. Positional
      2. Muscular
      3. Psychological disorder

tion may be defined as symptomatic excessive translation of the humeral head on the glenoid during shoulder motion. Harryman and associates[3] and Lippitt and associates[4] have demonstrated that shoulder laxity varies widely between individuals, and also that there is overlap in joint translation between those with asymptomatic shoulders and those with recurrent instability. Thus, it is crucial to keep in mind that the diagnosis of instability implies *symptoms* associated with excessive joint translations, and not merely laxity that appears to be greater than "normal."

With respect to direction, glenohumeral instability may be anterior, posterior, inferior, or combinations of these. When the subluxation or dislocation occurs in only one direction, it is termed unidirectional. Thomas and Matsen[5] have stressed the importance of distinguishing traumatic unidirectional cases (TUBS) from those with atraumatic multidirectional instability (AMBRI). Patients with multidirectional instability typically manifest signs of generalized ligamentous laxity, in addition to shoulder instability in all three directions—anterior, posterior, and inferior.[5,6] Others have recognized that there is another set of patients with an intermediate degree of instability, especially an inferior component in addition to an anterior or posterior direction.[7-9] Pollock and Bigliani[9] have termed this group bidirectional (anterior and inferior, or posterior and inferior). This type of instability appears to be more frequently seen in overhead athletes, perhaps because of the nature of the repetitive forces involved with overhead sports activities, which may stretch out the anterior and inferior capsular restraints. Interestingly, several authors have noted that patients with posterior glenohumeral instability often also have lesser degrees of inferior and/or anterior subluxation (ie, bidirectional or multidirectional types, rather than unidirectional). Establishing the direction of the instability and, in cases of instability in more than one direction, the primary direction and the direction of all lesser components of the instability, is essential in planning a successful strategy for treating the problem, particularly when surgical repair is contemplated. As Neer and Foster[6] have pointed out, failure to correct the instability fully can exacerbate the instability in the direction left unaddressed.

Concerning etiology, glenohumeral instability traditionally had been divided into traumatic and atraumatic types.[10] Neer has added the category of acquired instability to this classification.[11,12] This type of instability results from repetitive microtrauma (overuse) to the glenohumeral joint, such as that associated with pitching a baseball or swimming. Patients frequently present with a history that implicates several factors in the pathogenesis of their shoulder instability. A young swimmer with a great degree of congenital ligamentous laxity, for example, may develop symptomatic instability after swimming for several years (repetitive microtrauma) or may not become symptomatic until after a traumatic event. The etiologic categories often become blurred, particularly in young athletes who participate in overhead sports activities. These patients demonstrate that overlap between etiologic categories rather than only two or three discrete groups, may exist in a clinical population. Glenohumeral instability can be thought of as a spectrum ranging from relatively atraumatic multidirectional instability to bidirectional instability, which is often associated with repetitive microtrauma, to unidirectional instability that is frequently a result of trauma (Fig. 19). Overlap in direction, etiology, and degree will exist in this continuum of shoulder instability, emphasizing the need for careful diagnosis in each case.

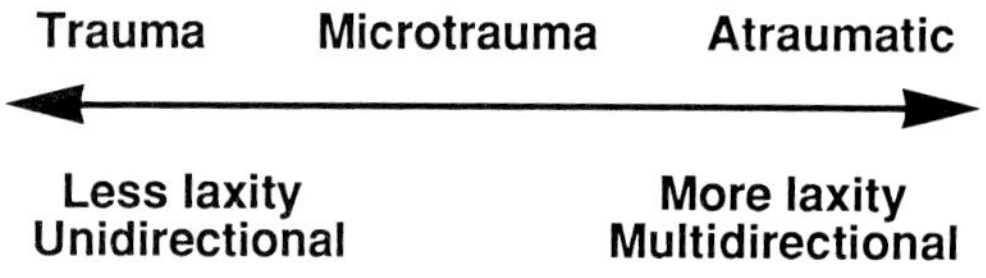

Trauma   Microtrauma   Atraumatic

$\longleftrightarrow$

**Less laxity   More laxity
Unidirectional   Multidirectional**

FIGURE 19
The spectrum of instability.

The issue of volition is also addressed in the classification of glenohumeral instability. The instability can be voluntary, in which case the patient can bring about or demonstrate an episode of subluxation or dislocation at will, or involuntary, in which case the episodes are completely outside the control of the patient. Voluntary instability is more commonly seen in cases of posterior and multidirectional instability. Rowe and associates[13] have pointed out that within the group of voluntary dislocators is a subset of patients with significant emotional or psychological problems. These patients use their shoulder instability as a means of getting attention. Identification of this type of volitional instability is crucial, because these patients will frustrate efforts at treatment if the underlying psychological problem is not also treated.[6,13] Many patients with voluntary instability, however, do not have a psychological disorder. These patients are able to demonstrate the instability by placing the shoulder in positions that cause subluxation (eg, for posterior instability in combined flexion to 90°, adduction, and internal rotation). This positional type of voluntary instability has benefited from surgical stabilization.[14,15] In a third subgroup, patients in whom selective muscle activation results in subluxation or dislocation, the voluntary component may be an unconscious behavioral tic. This muscular type of voluntary instability is thought to respond better to biofeedback techniques.[16] The identification of a voluntary component, as well as its precise characterization, is crucial in classifying and treating glenohumeral instability.

EVALUATION

A careful history and physical examination are the most important tools in evaluating a shoulder for suspected glenohumeral instability. In cases of acute unreduced dislocations, radiographs will demonstrate the diagnosis; however, in more subtle forms of instability, or in the period between episodes of instability, the surgeon must rely most heavily on the history and physical examination to make the correct diagnosis. In these cases, radiographs may provide corroborating evidence for glenohumeral instability or for a particular type of instability, but they also may be normal. More sophisticated radiographic imaging techniques, such as CT, computed arthrotomography (arthro-CT), and MRI, may occasionally add useful information, but they are not necessary in the routine evaluation of glenohumeral instability. Examination of the shoulder under anesthesia and/or by arthroscopy can be helpful in some difficult cases to confirm the diagnosis of instability and to more precisely determine the direction(s). These techniques, however, are reserved for unusual cases, in which the history and physical examination suggest glenohumeral instability but doubt remains about the diagnosis and appropriate treatment.

HISTORY

A thorough investigation of the onset of symptoms is quite helpful in correctly diagnosing and classifying glenohumeral instability. The physician should inquire about the circumstances surrounding the first episode of dislocation or subluxation, to learn whether there was an episode of major trauma (eg, a wrenching of the arm during a football tackle or a wrestling takedown), trivial trauma (eg, throwing a ball or swimming certain strokes), or no trauma at all (eg, merely reaching overhead). The extent or degree of the initial injury must be explored. Was there a locked dislocation, which required a reduction by a physician or another person (teammate, athletic trainer, or family member), or could the shoulder be self-reduced, as in a transient subluxation? If there was a locked dislocation that required treatment by a physician, are radiographs from the initial episode available? These radiographs would, of course, provide documentation of the diagnosis of instability and would demonstrate the major direction of the instability. Similar inquiries about the circumstances of subsequent episodes should also be made, to learn how many such episodes have occurred, how many have required reduction by another individual (versus spontaneous reduction), and whether the episodes are now occurring more easily (ie, with less force) and more frequently.

Knowing the position of the arm at the time of the initial episode and the direction of the forces placed on it at the time of the initial injury can be helpful in establishing the direction of the instability, especially when injury radiographs are not available. Often the patient will not be able to remember the exact mechanism of injury, particularly when there has been a sudden impact to the arm. The patient more likely will be able to relate which arm positions and activities reproduce the symptoms or actually result in episodes of recurrent instability. Pain and apprehension (a feeling that the shoulder is about to sublux or dislocate) while using the shoulder in a combined position of abduction, external rotation, and extension suggest instability that is primarily anterior. Symptoms with the arm in a relatively flexed, adducted, and internally rotated position suggest posterior instability.

The physician should also inquire about prior treatment that has been provided for this problem. The type and arm position of immobilization, the length of immobilization, and the nature of any rehabilitative program that has been undertaken should be documented. If the patient has had a prior failed attempt at surgical repair of the instability, it is important to investigate the symptoms and nature of the episodes both before and after the failed repair. A shoulder that once dislocated anteriorly, for example, may now sublux posteriorly after an excessively tight anterior repair. Thus the qualitative nature of the instability may change after a surgical intervention, and a thorough history will provide this information. A prior operative report also should be obtained to help evaluate what was done at the initial surgery. These patients often present with a complex clinical picture, with multiple factors contributing to the failure, and require an especially careful evaluation before proceeding with further treatment.

After addressing issues surrounding the prior episodes of instability and earlier attempts at treatment, the physician should then inquire about symptoms that the patient is presently experiencing. Patients with instability will often complain that the arm "slips out and then back in" with certain activities. This description of a sensation of subluxation followed by a sensation of spontaneous reduction provides strong evidence for a diagnosis of glenohumeral instability. In another subgroup of patients with this problem, however, pain is the major complaint rather than a feeling of instability. Frequently, patients with instability (especially dislocators) experience pain only during episodes of frank instability and for a brief period (a few days or weeks) after the event. Others will complain of pain only with particular arm positions or activities, while a third group will experience a constant ache. Knowing only the location of the pain rarely allows the physician to diagnose instability. Although anterior shoulder pain is often associated with anterior glenohumeral instability, especially in younger athletes, it is by no means unique to this diagnosis. Pain in the anterior shoulder may be present in a number of other shoulder disorders, particularly with subacromial inflammation or impingement. Furthermore, patients with anterior instability may complain of posterior shoulder pain, perhaps due to a secondary tendinitis of the posterior rotator cuff or to inflammation of the synovial joint lining with episodes of subluxation.

The location of pain in the context of arm position or a provocative activity, however, may be more helpful in clarifying the diagnosis of instability. In throwing athletes, for example, symptoms occurring mainly during the cocking phase of the throw often indicate an anterior instability, while those occurring primarily during the follow-through often point to a posterior subluxation. Symptoms that occur while carrying a heavy object, such as a suitcase, with the arm at the side usually suggest that a component of inferior instability is present. Thus, placing symptoms into a particular context can assist in determining the direction(s) of an instability.

Other symptoms, such as popping or clicking in the shoulder, may suggest glenohumeral instability; however, these may be associated with other types of pathology, such as superior labral (SLAP) lesions.[17] Glenohumeral instability may also present as a "dead arm syndrome" as described by Rowe and Zarins.[18] In this presentation, patients with anterior subluxations experience sudden "paralyzing pain," and briefly lose control of the arm when it is in the cocking position.[18] Similar neurologic complaints may be seen in patients with inferior subluxation when they carry heavy objects in the involved arm. Often these neurologic symptoms are localized chiefly in the ulnar aspect of the forearm and hand. Other disorders, such as cervical radiculopathy, mild brachial plexus injuries, and thoracic outlet syndrome, also may present in this manner and should be considered when neurologic complaints are significant. Glenohumeral instability and thoracic outlet syndrome may also co-exist in the same patient and may require separate treatment for each problem.[19]

Inquiries must also be made about functional losses due to the shoulder instability. Some patients will have disrupted function only during rare episodes of dislocation. More commonly, the instability will interfere with high demand activities, such as throwing a baseball or serving a tennis ball. In these activities, the arm assumes the extreme provocative positions that elicit pain or a sensation of instability in the athlete. Others will have symptoms during the performance of routine activities of daily living or even at rest. The amount of disability and the motivation and activity level of the patient must be assessed, especially when considering a surgical repair. Patients with milder symptoms or those with symptoms only during particular sports activities may choose to modify their activities, rather than undergo reconstructive surgery. Those with greater disability and those who desire to remain active in their sport are more likely to choose surgical repair if nonsurgical treatment fails.

Finally, the issue of voluntary control over the instability must be addressed by the physician in evaluating patients with glenohumeral instability. The patient should be questioned about voluntary dislocation during childhood or adolescence, either as a behavioral tic or a party trick. The physician must also be alert for signs that the voluntary instability may reflect an underlying emotional problem, as previously discussed. In these cases, the patient is not likely to admit the true motivation for producing subluxations and dislocations. Nonverbal cues, such as the manner in which the patient relates to the parents during the interview and examination, can be quite helpful in this respect. Recognizing the presence of a volitional component and accurately clarifying which type of voluntary instability it represents will influence determination of appropriate treatment.

PHYSICAL EXAMINATION

A careful physical examination is the other crucial tool in evaluating the patient with suspected glenohumeral instability. Both shoulders are examined, in order to compare them with respect to laxity, strength, range of motion, and the presence or absence of symptoms with provocative tests for stability. It is useful to begin by examining the asymptomatic side, as this will indicate the normal amount of laxity for that patient. Moreover, since the examination of the contralateral shoulder will usually not elicit symptoms, it may help the patient relax during performance of similar maneuvers on the symptomatic shoulder. The physician should evaluate the contralateral shoulder with respect to laxity in the anterior, posterior, and inferior directions, keeping in mind that many patients with multidirectional instability will exhibit bilaterally loose shoulders. Other signs of generalized ligamentous laxity are also sought—hyperextension of the elbow, hyperextension of the metacarpophalangeal joints, the ability to touch the abducted thumb to the ipsilateral forearm (thumb-to-forearm test), and hypermobility of the patella. Particularly when the symptomatic shoulder is difficult to examine adequately because of pain and guarding by the patient, the results of tests on the contralateral shoulder and other joints may help to uncover an instability that is multidirectional.

The physician then examines the symptomatic shoulder. Inspection of the shoulder usually fails to demonstrate atrophy of the deltoid or spinati muscles. Occasionally with a traumatic dislocation in a young patient, and with increasing incidence over 40 years of age, there will be an accompanying nerve injury and/or a tear of the rotator cuff (posterior mechanism).[20] Injury to the axillary nerve may result in atrophy of the deltoid and a persistent inability to raise the arm overhead, even after the acute period of injury. The presence of a concomitant rotator cuff tear can result in atrophy of the supraspinatus and infraspinatus, as well as persistent weakness. Mild scapular winging may occasionally be seen in cases of recurrent posterior glenohumeral instability and may represent an attempt to prevent the shoulder from subluxating posteriorly by reorienting the position of the scapula. More impressive degrees of scapular winging should prompt the examiner to consider possible injury to the spinal accessory or long thoracic nerves.

Palpation of the shoulder must include the sternoclavicular and acromioclavicular joints, as well as the glenohumeral region. A tender acromioclavicular joint may be the source of the patient's symptoms and should not be neglected because the examiner is distracted by an asymptomatically lax glenohumeral joint. Patients with anterior glenohumeral instability will often have tenderness with palpation over the anterior shoulder; however, this finding is nonspecific and is seen with many shoulder conditions, particularly with subacromial impingement. Tenderness over the posterior glenohumeral joint line is frequently seen in patients with posterior instability, but this too is a nonspecific finding.

The range of motion of the symptomatic shoulder is measured and compared with that of the contralateral shoulder. Typically, patients with glenohumeral instability will have a full range of motion. The patient with anterior instability may be apprehensive or even guard during measurement of external rotation with the arm abducted to 90°. Discomfort may also result from full external rotation with the arm at the side.[12] In patients who have undergone failed instability surgery, the symptomatic shoulder may have limitations in motion, particularly in external rotation after an anterior tightening of the shoulder. In this group, combinations of stiffness in certain planes with instability in other planes are not uncommon, and motion and stability must be carefully examined in multiple arm positions.

The stability of the affected shoulder is then assessed by carrying out a number of provocative maneuvers designed to reproduce the patient's instability symptoms. The sulcus test is used to identify an inferior instability component in a bidirectionally or multidirectionally unstable shoulder. This test is first performed by pulling downward on the arm, which is positioned at the patient's side (Fig. 20, *left*). The maneuver is then repeated with the arm abducted to 90°, as the examiner places a downward force on the proximal humerus (Fig. 20, *right*).[6,21] The patient's shoulder muscles must be relaxed during the maneuvers, in order to successfully interpret the test results. It is usually helpful to perform this test prior to other provocative tests that may stimulate pain and reflex muscle guarding and prevent adequate assessment of a sulcus.

Laxity in the anterior and posterior directions is then measured by a drawer test or "shift and load" test.[22] With the patient in a sitting position, the physician grasps the proximal humerus between the thumb and index fingers, with the patient's arm positioned at the side. The humeral head is pushed into the center of the glenoid fossa to ensure its reduction to the neutral position at the start of the test (ie, "loaded"). A manual force is then exerted in an anterior direction and the translation is measured. The humeral head is then recentered and a posterior drawer test is performed. This testing can also be repeated with the patient supine. Relaxation of the shoulder muscles is essential to gain useful information about the degree of laxity.

The anterior apprehension test (crank test) is performed next, with the patient in a sitting position. The arm is placed in 90° of abduction with the elbow flexed to 90°. The examiner progressively rotates the arm externally and extends it with one hand, while exerting an anteriorly direct-

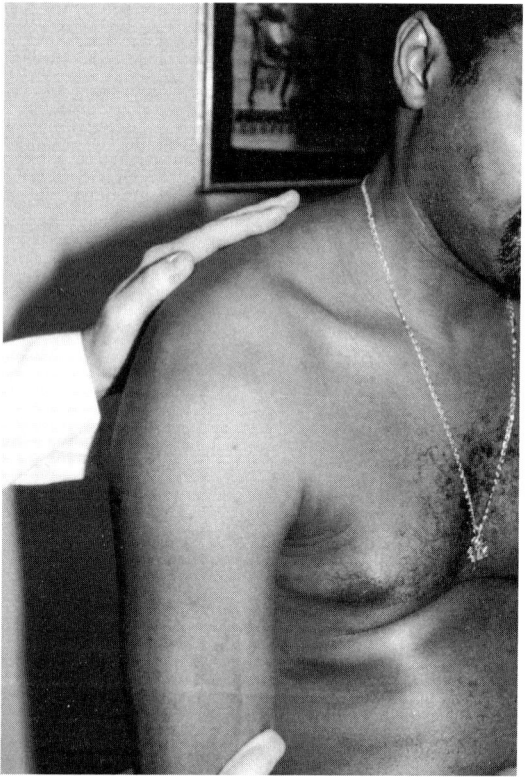
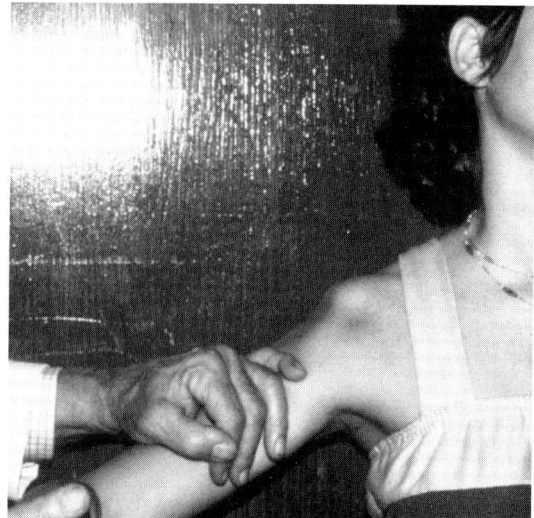

FIGURE 20

Left, The sulcus test is first performed by pulling downward on the patient's arm, which is positioned at the patient's side. A dimple or sulcus is seen beneath the acromion in a positive test. **Right,** The test is then repeated with the arm in greater abduction, because different ligamentous stabilizers are primary with different arm positions. Again, a sulcus sign is seen beneath the acromion in a positive test.

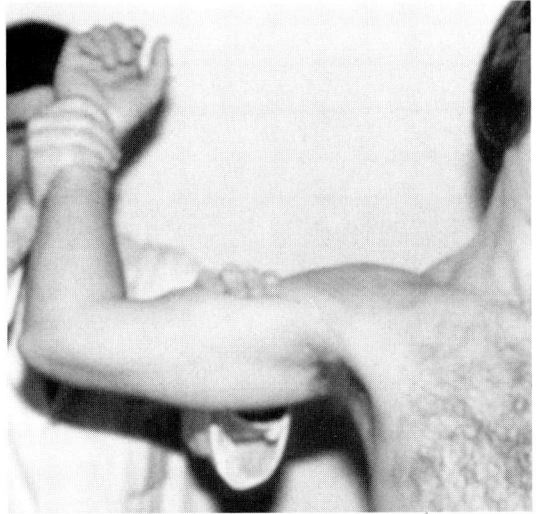

FIGURE 21

Anterior apprehension test. The arm is placed in 90° of abduction with the elbow flexed to 90°. The examiner progressively extends and rotates the arm externally with one hand, while exerting an anteriorly directed force on the humeral head with the other. Patients with anterior instability will experience true apprehension (a feeling of imminent subluxation or dislocation) with this maneuver.

ed force on the humeral head (Fig. 21). Patients with anterior instability will manifest true apprehension (a feeling of imminent subluxation or dislocation) with this maneuver. If pain alone is elicited, a number of other painful shoulder conditions must be considered, especially subacromial impingement. A subacromial lidocaine injection can be useful in distinguishing between these two entities; however, both may be present in the same shoulder in a young athlete.[23] The relocation maneuver may be used to help differentiate between glenohumeral instability and impingement.[24] This test is performed with the patient in a supine position (Fig. 22). The anterior apprehension maneuver is carried out while pushing anteriorly on the humeral head. The test is then repeated with a posteriorly directed force applied by the examiner over the anterior aspect of the humeral head, to stabilize it in a reduced position. If the patient's symptoms are eliminated with this second maneuver, the diagnosis of subluxation is favored. It has recently been demonstrated, however, that this test is much more specific for instability when only true apprehension and not merely pain is considered a positive response.[25]

A posterior stress test is then performed to evaluate whether there is a posterior component of instability. In this test, the patient is in the sitting position. The examiner stabilizes the scapula with one hand and with the other exerts a posteriorly directed force on the humerus, which is flexed to 90°, adducted, and internally rotated (Fig. 23). A positive test produces subluxation with pain or a sensation that reproduces the uncomfortable feeling the patient experiences during an episode of instability. Painless transla-

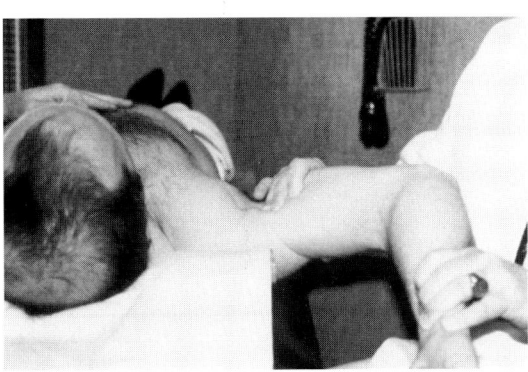

FIGURE 22

Relocation test. The anterior apprehension test is first performed with the patient supine. Next, this maneuver of progressive external rotation and extension is repeated, while the examiner also applies a posteriorly directed force over the humeral head. If the sensation of apprehension is eliminated during this second maneuver, the diagnosis of anterior instability is supported.

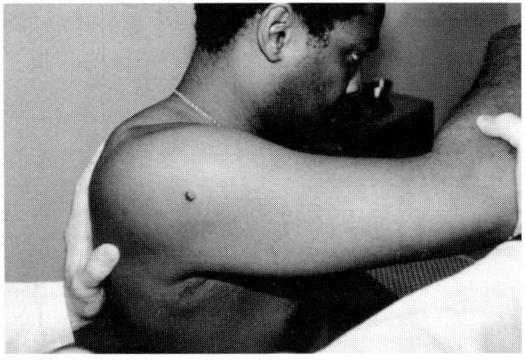

FIGURE 23

Posterior stress test. The examiner stabilizes the scapula with one hand and with the other exerts a posteriorly directed force on the arm, which is flexed to 90°, adducted, and internally rotated. A positive test produces subluxation with pain or reproduces the patient's symptoms that are experienced during episodes of subluxation. This test is very helpful for diagnosing posterior glenohumeral instability.

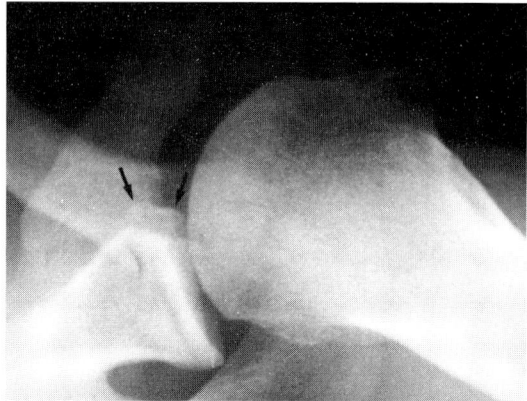

FIGURE 24
The axillary radiograph is helpful in demonstrating associated fractures or erosion of the glenoid rim (arrows) in a patient with glenohumeral instability.

tion of the humeral head over the glenoid rim posteriorly indicates laxity, but is not sufficient for a diagnosis of posterior instability. The posterior stress test differs from the anterior apprehension test in that it usually produces pain rather than true apprehension. The patient will usually allow the test to be completed, although it does reproduce the discomfort associated with an episode of instability in nearly all patients with posterior glenohumeral instability.

RADIOGRAPHIC EVALUATION

The radiographic evaluation after an acute episode of trauma to the shoulder in which a dislocation is suspected ideally includes three orthogonal views of the glenohumeral joint. This "trauma series" includes anteroposterior and lateral views in the plane of the scapula and an axillary view.[26] These views will allow accurate determination of the direction of the dislocation and will avoid the trap of missing a locked posterior dislocation that may be difficult to diagnose from anteroposterior views alone.[26-28] The Velpeau axillary view, described by Bloom and Obata,[29] is an especially advantageous axillary radiograph after trauma. With this view, the arm remains immobilized in a sling, thus ensuring less discomfort for the patient and preventing displacement of associated fractures of the proximal humerus during the process of obtaining radiographs. The axillary radiograph will also be helpful in demonstrating associated fractures or erosions of the glenoid rim (Fig. 24).

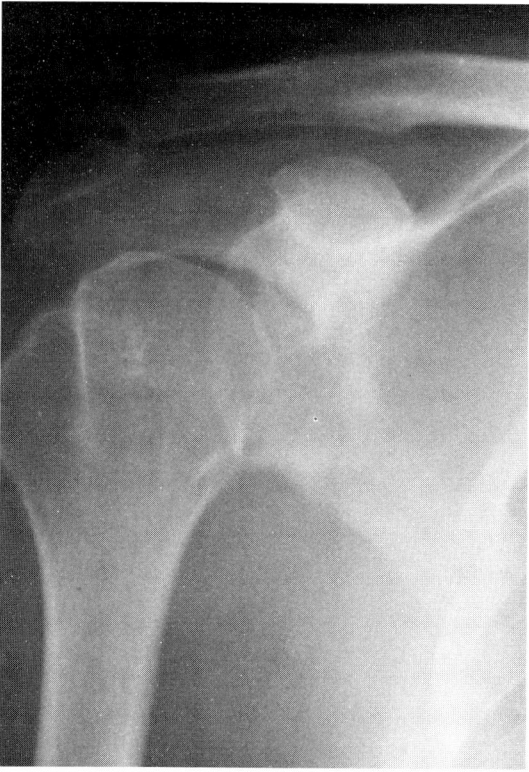

FIGURE 25
The anteroposterior radiograph of the shoulder with the arm in internal rotation demonstrates the posterolateral impression defect of the humeral head (Hill-Sachs lesion) seen commonly after traumatic dislocations.

Routine radiographs for evaluating the shoulder in the absence of trauma often include anteroposterior views in different positions of arm rotation (external, neutral, and internal), a lateral view of the scapula ("Y view"), and an axillary view. Warren[30] has proposed an "instability series" to include a true anteroposterior view of the shoulder with the arm in internal rotation (Fig. 25), a West Point axillary view,[31] and a Stryker notch view (Fig. 26).[32] In the West Point axillary view, the patient is prone with the shoulder abducted 90° and internally rotated. The X-ray beam is centered at the axilla and is directed downward 25° and medially 25°. It allows detection of even subtle bony changes or erosions of the anterior glenoid rim. The Stryker notch view is performed with the patient supine and the arm flexed so that the hand rests behind the patient's head. The X-ray beam is tilted 10° cephalic and

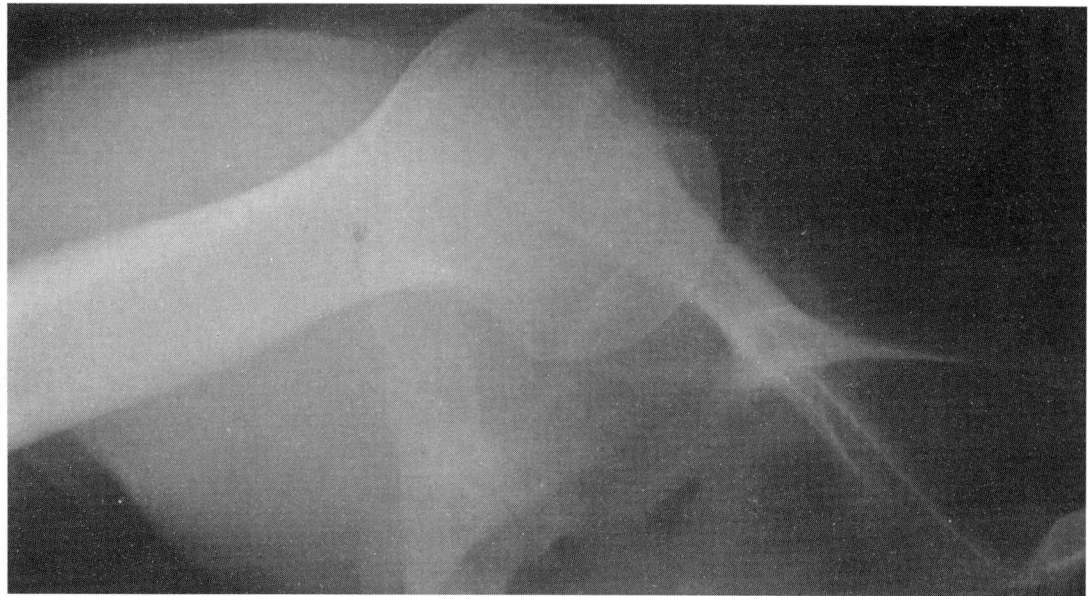

FIGURE 26
The Stryker notch view also shows the hatchet-like defect in the posterolateral humeral head (Hill-Sachs lesion).

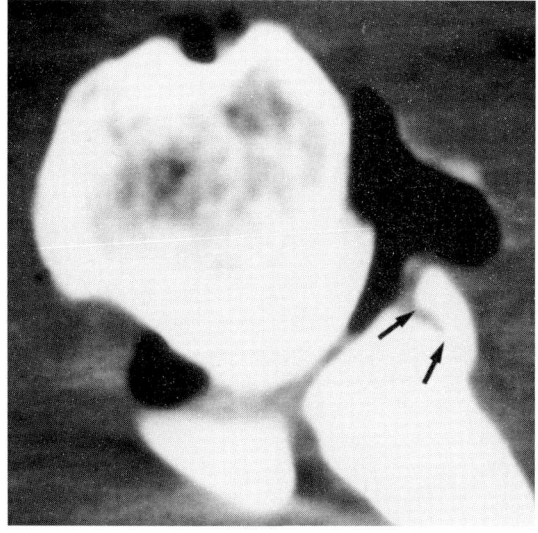

FIGURE 27
CT arthrography can delineate and quantify bony glenoid lesions, such as anterior rim fractures (black arrows). This imaging technique can also demonstrate soft-tissue lesions, such as labral detachment and excessive capsular volume.

aimed toward the coracoid. This view allows accurate identification of a Hill-Sachs lesion. The apical oblique view is another helpful view, par-

ticularly in evaluating erosions or fractures of the anterior glenoid rim.[33] Stress radiographs in the anteroposterior and axillary planes have been used in the past to demonstrate instability,[34,35] but are presently rarely employed.

More sophisticated imaging modalities also may be used to evaluate glenohumeral instability, but are generally reserved for selected cases. CT can accurately demonstrate the size of associated glenoid fractures and impression fractures of the humeral head in locked posterior fracture-dislocations. When the axillary radiographs suggest abnormalities of glenoid development (eg, hypoplasia) or version, the CT scan can help delineate these abnormalities. Because bony pathology is usually not implicated in the etiology of glenohumeral instability, a CT scan is necessary only rarely. CT arthrography can demonstrate soft-tissue pathology, such as irregularities or detachment of the labrum and excessive capsular redundancy (Fig. 27).[36-40] These scans have been shown to correlate quite well with surgical findings in several studies.[37,38,40] MRI also has been used to evaluate glenohumeral instability. Several studies have found MRI to be quite accurate in evaluating lesions of the anterior glenoid labrum.[41-43] Legan and associates,[43] however, have found MRI to be less successful in detecting posteroinferior labral

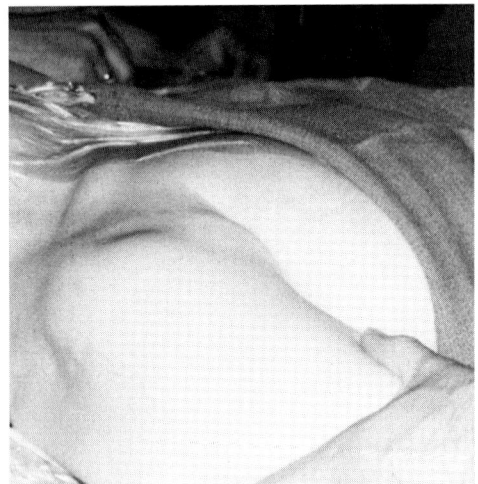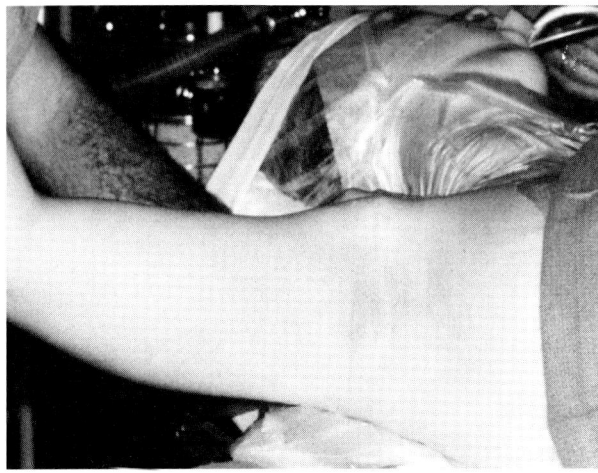

FIGURE 28
Left and **right,** An examination under anesthesia is helpful in evaluating selected cases of suspected glenohumeral instability. The EUA allows confirmation of the diagnosis, as well as clarification of the predominant direction and lesser components of the instability. Stability is tested in all three directions (anterior, posterior, and inferior), using a number of different positions of abduction and rotation.

pathology, perhaps because of capsular redundancy in this region. Green and Christensen[44] have suggested that MRI is not useful in surgical planning for most patients with obvious anterior shoulder instability, while Press and associates[45] concluded that at present CT arthrography remains a superior diagnostic procedure for evaluating glenohumeral instability. When an associated tear of the rotator cuff is suspected after an acute dislocation in a patient over 40 years of age, MRI would certainly be useful. All of the special imaging studies are expensive, however, and are certainly not recommended for routine use in the evaluation of glenohumeral instability.

EXAMINATION UNDER ANESTHESIA
A number of authors have pointed out the value of an examination under anesthesia (EUA) in evaluating cases of subtle instability.[21,30,46] The EUA may help to clarify the diagnosis in patients in whom instability is suspected yet the diagnosis remains uncertain due to limitations in the office history and physical examination. In heavily muscled athletes or patients with considerable shoulder pain, the examiner may not be able to elicit helpful information from the physical examination because of muscle guarding. The EUA can be used to confirm the diagnosis in these patients, especially when surgical reconstruction is planned. The

predominant direction of the instability, as well as lesser components of the instability, can be clarified through the EUA. It is unusual, however, for the findings on EUA to contradict the diagnosis that has been established through the history and physical examination.

During the performance of the EUA, it is important to establish a frame of reference so that the reduction of a posterior subluxation is not mistaken for a subluxation of the humeral head anteriorly.[21,30,46] Bony anatomic landmarks, such as the coracoid anteriorly and the posterolateral acromion, are used to provide this frame of reference. Before each maneuver, the humeral head must be centered on the glenoid to prevent mistaking a reduction for a subluxation in the opposite direction. Stability is tested in all three directions (anterior, posterior, and inferior), using a number of different arm positions of abduction and rotation (Fig. 28).[46] Documentation of the findings of EUA using fluoroscopy has been reported,[35] but this is usually not necessary for an experienced examiner.

An arthroscopic examination may be added to the EUA, in order to provide additional pathoanatomic information about the instability. Through arthroscopy, anatomic lesions such as a detached anteroinferior glenoid labrum, a Hill-Sachs lesion, and excessive capsular redundancy can be directly visualized.[47-49] Subtle signs of occult instability, such as labral fraying or wear, can be detected and the rotator cuff and biceps complex can be evaluated. This is particularly helpful in overhead throwing athletes, who frequently present with an overlap syndrome (ie, instability with secondary subacromial impingement)[23] and superior labral pathology (SLAP lesions).[17] The information gained from the arthroscopy can confirm the suspected diagnosis and may also help determine if the patient is a suitable candidate for arthroscopic stabilization. The use of EUA and arthroscopy can provide useful information in selected cases of glenohumeral instability. As is the case with specialized imaging techniques, however, these tools are not necessary for routine diagnosis of glenohumeral instability.

REFERENCES

1. McLaughlin HL: Posterior dislocation of the shoulder. *J Bone Joint Surg* 1952;34A:584-590.

2. Hawkins RJ, Neer CS II, Pianta RM, et al: Locked posterior dislocation of the shoulder. *J Bone Joint Surg* 1987;69A:9-18.

3. Harryman DT II, Sidles JA, Harris SL, et al: Laxity of the normal glenohumeral joint: A quantitative in vivo assessment. *J Shoulder Elbow Surg* 1992;1:66-76.

4. Lippitt SB, Harris SL, Harryman DT II, et al: In vivo quantification of the laxity of normal and unstable glenohumeral joints. *J Shoulder Elbow Surg* 1994;3:215-223.

5. Thomas SC, Matsen FA III: An approach to the repair of avulsion of the glenohumeral ligaments in the management of traumatic anterior glenohumeral instability. *J Bone Joint Surg* 1989;71A:506-513.

6. Neer CS II, Foster CR: Inferior capsular shift for involuntary inferior and multidirectional instability of the shoulder: A preliminary report. *J Bone Joint Surg* 1980;62A:897-908.

7. Altchek DW, Warren RF, Skyhar MJ, et al: T-plasty modification of the Bankart procedure for multidirectional instability of the anterior and inferior types. *J Bone Joint Surg* 1991;73A:105-112.

8. Bigliani LU, Kurzweil PR, Schwartzbach CC, et al: Inferior capsular shift procedure for anterior/inferior shoulder instability in athletes. *Am J Sports Med* 1994;22:578-584.

9. Pollock RG, Bigliani LU: Recurrent posterior shoulder instability: Diagnosis and treatment. *Clin Orthop* 1993;291:85-96.

10. Rowe CR: Prognosis in dislocations of the shoulder. *J Bone Joint Surg* 1956;38A:957-977.

11. Neer CS II: Recent concepts in dislocation and subluxation, in Takagishi N (ed): *The Shoulder: Proceedings of the Third International Conference on Surgery of the Shoulder.* Tokyo, Japan, Professional Postgraduate Services, 1987, pp 7-12.

12. Neer CS II (ed): *Shoulder Reconstruction.* Philadelphia, PA, WB Saunders, 1990.

13. Rowe CR, Pierce DS, Clark JG: Voluntary dislocation of the shoulder: A preliminary report on a clinical, electromyographic, and psychiatric study of twenty-six patients. *J Bone Joint Surg* 1973;55A:445-460.

14. Fronek J, Warren RF, Bowen M: Posterior subluxation of the glenohumeral joint. *J Bone Joint Surg* 1989;71A:205-216

15. Bigliani LU, Pollock RG, Endrizzi DP, et al: Surgical repair of posterior instability of the shoulder: Long-term results. *Orthop Trans* 1993;17:75-76.

16. Beall MS Jr, Diefenbach G, Allen A: Electromyographic biofeedback in the treatment of voluntary posterior instability of the shoulder. *Am J Sports Med* 1987;15:175-178.

17. Snyder SJ, Karzel RP, Del Pizzo W, et al: SLAP lesions of the shoulder. *Arthroscopy* 1990;6:274-279.

18. Rowe CR, Zarins B: Recurrent transient subluxation of the shoulder. *J Bone Joint Surg* 1981;63A:863-872.

19. Leffert RD, Gumley G: The relationship between dead arm syndrome and thoracic outlet syndrome. *Clin Orthop* 1987;223:20-31.

20. McLaughlin HL, MacLellan DI: Recurrent anterior dislocation of the shoulder: II. A comparative study. *J Trauma* 1967;7:191-201.

21. Neer CS II: Involuntary inferior and multidirectional instability of the shoulder: Etiology, recognition and treatment, in Stauffer ES (ed): American Academy of Orthopaedic Surgeons *Instructional Course Lectures Volume XXXIV.* St. Louis, MO, CV Mosby, 1985, pp 232-238.

22. Hawkins RJ, Bokor DJ: Clinical evaluation of shoulder problems, in Rockwood CA Jr, Matsen FA III (eds): *The Shoulder.* Philadelphia, PA, WB Saunders, 1990, pp 149-177.

23. Jobe FW, Kvitne RS, Giangarra CE: Shoulder pain in the overhand or throwing athlete: The relationship of anterior instability and rotator cuff impingement. *Orthop Rev* 1989;18:963-975.

24. Jobe FW, Tibone JE, Jobe CM, et al: The shoulder in sports, in Rockwood CA Jr, Matsen FA III (eds): *The Shoulder*. Philadelphia, PA, WB Saunders, 1990, vol 2, 961-990.

25. Speer KP, Hannafin JA, Altchek DW, et al: An evaluation of the shoulder relocation test. *Am J Sports Med* 1994;22:177-183.

26. Neer CS II: Displaced proximal humeral fractures: I. Classification and evaluation. *J Bone Joint Surg* 1970;52A:1077-1089.

27. Rockwood CA Jr, Szalay EA, Curtis RJ Jr, et al: X-ray evaluation of shoulder problems, in Rockwood CA Jr, Matsen FA III (eds): *The Shoulder*. Philadelphia, PA, WB Saunders, 1990, pp 178-207.

28. Neviaser RJ: Radiologic assessment of the shoulder: Plain and arthrographic. *Orthop Clin North Am* 1987;18:343-349.

29. Bloom MH, Obata WG: Diagnosis of posterior dislocation of the shoulder with use of Velpeau axillary and angle-up roentgenographic views. *J Bone Joint Surg* 1967;49A:943-949.

30. Warren RF: Subluxation of the shoulder in athletes. *Clin Sports Med* 1983;2:339-354.

31. Rokous JR, Feagin JA, Abbott HG: Modified axillary roentgenogram: A useful adjunct in the diagnosis of recurrent instability of the shoulder. *Clin Orthop* 1972;82:84-86.

32. Hall RH, Isaac F, Booth CR: Dislocations of the shoulder with special reference to accompanying small fractures. *J Bone Joint Surg* 1959;41A:489-494.

33. Garth WP Jr, Slappey CE, Ochs CW: Roentgenographic demonstration of instability of the shoulder: The apical oblique projection. A technical note. *J Bone Joint Surg* 1984;66A:1450-1453.

34. Adler H, Lohmann B: The stability of the shoulder joint in stress radiography. *Arch Orthop Trauma Surg* 1984;103:83-84.

35. Norris TR: Diagnostic techniques for shoulder instability, in Stauffer ES (ed): American Academy of Orthopaedic Surgeons *Instructional Course Lectures Volume XXXIV*. St. Louis, MO, CV Mosby, 1985, pp 239-257.

36. Danzig L, Resnick D, Greenway G: Evaluation of unstable shoulders by computed tomography: A preliminary study. *Am J Sports Med* 1982;10:138-141.

37. Rafii M, Firooznia H, Golimbu C, et al: CT arthrography of capsular structures of the shoulder. *Am J Roentgenol* 1986;146:361-367.

38. Singson RD, Feldman F, Bigliani L: CT arthrographic patterns in recurrent glenohumeral instability. *Am J Roentgenol* 1987;149:749-753.

39. Randelli M, Odella F, Gambrioli PL: Clinical experience with double contrast medium computerised tomography (arthro-CT) in instability of the shoulder. *Ital J Orthop Traumatol* 1986;12:151-158.

40. Kinnard P, Tricoire JL, Levesque R, et al: Assessment of the unstable shoulder by computed arthrography. A preliminary report. *Am J Sports Med* 1983;11:157-159.

41. Iannotti JP, Zlatkin MB, Esterhai JL, et al: Magnetic resonance imaging of the shoulder: Sensitivity, specificity, and predictive value. *J Bone Joint Surg* 1991;73A:17-29.

42. Seeger LL, Gold RH, Bassett LW: Shoulder instability: Evaluation with MR imaging. *Radiology* 1988;168:695-697.

43. Legan JM, Burkhard TK, Goff WB II, et al: Tears of the glenoid labrum: MR imaging of 88 arthroscopically confirmed cases. *Radiology* 1991;179:241-246.

44. Green MR, Christensen KP: Magnetic resonance imaging of the glenoid labrum in anterior shoulder instability. *Am J Sports Med* 1994;22:493-498.

45. Press JA, Zuckerman JD, Cuomo F: Imaging of shoulder instability. *Oper Tech Sports Med* 1993;1:256-267.

46. Cofield RH, Irving JF: Evaluation and classification of shoulder instability: With special reference to examination under anesthesia. *Clin Orthop* 1987;223:32-43.

47. McGlynn FJ, Caspari RB: Arthroscopic findings in the subluxating shoulder. *Clin Orthop* 1984;183:173-178.

48. Cofield RH: Arthroscopy of the shoulder. *Mayo Clin Proc* 1983;58:501-508.

49. Baker CL, Uribe JW, Whitman C: Arthroscopic evaluation of acute initial anterior shoulder dislocations. *Am J Sports Med* 1990;18:25-28.

ACUTE TRAUMATIC ANTERIOR DISLOCATION OF THE SHOULDER

ROBERT A. ARCIERO, MD

ACUTE TRAUMATIC DISLOCATION

Acute anterior shoulder dislocations represent the most dramatic form of a shoulder instability event. A major traumatic event, such as a fall onto the shoulder or a collision, frequently precipitates the dislocation. One of the most common mechanisms of injury involves a force couple of humeral abduction and external rotation (Figs. 29 and 30), as would occur during arm tackling in football, blocking a shot in basketball, or traversing an overhead ladder on a military obstacle course. Although such injuries occur primarily in young athletes, any fall of sufficient magnitude with the arm in abduction and external rotation can cause a dislocation.

The patient typically presents in extreme pain with the arm at the side and with significant guarding. The normal contour of the deltoid and prominence of the acromion are lost. Because an anterior dislocation blocks the humerus from achieving complete internal rotation and abduction, motion is restricted. Careful neurologic and vascular examinations are important. Axillary nerve injuries are the most common nerve injury, with an incidence as high as 35%.[1] In the more elderly population with acquired atherosclerosis and vessel rigidity, axillary artery avulsions can occur after anterior dislocation.[2]

Three radiographs are required to fully evaluate the injury. The standard anteroposterior (AP) view, an axillary or modified axillary view (West Point view), and a transscapular lateral view[2-4] will permit identification of associated glenoid rim fractures (Fig. 31), Hill-Sachs lesions (posterolateral humeral head defects), and fractures of the greater tuberosity (Fig. 32). Importantly, these views will confirm that the dislocation is anterior rather than posterior.

Occasionally, when an athlete sustains an acute dislocation during a game, it may be reasonable to consider a gentle reduction on the field *prior to* obtaining radiographs. In this instance, it is frequently possible to perform the reduction within minutes of the dislocation before pain and muscle spasm develop.[2,5]

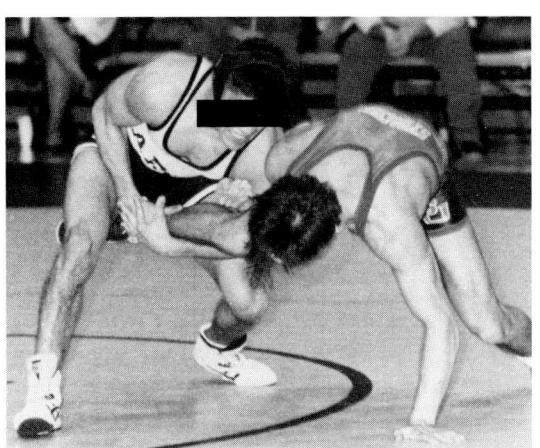

FIGURE 29
Force couple of abduction in external rotation being applied to the left shoulder of a wrestler.

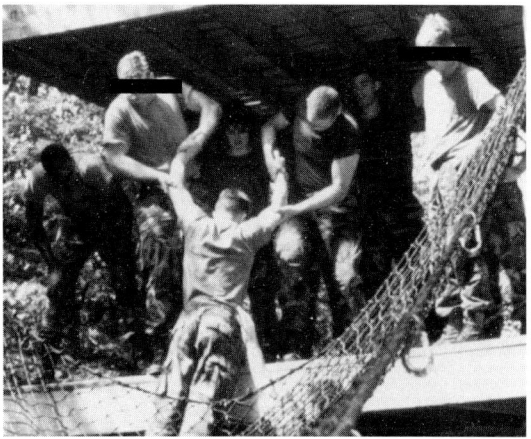

FIGURE 30
Abduction and external rotation stress applied to cadet in negotiating an obstacle course.

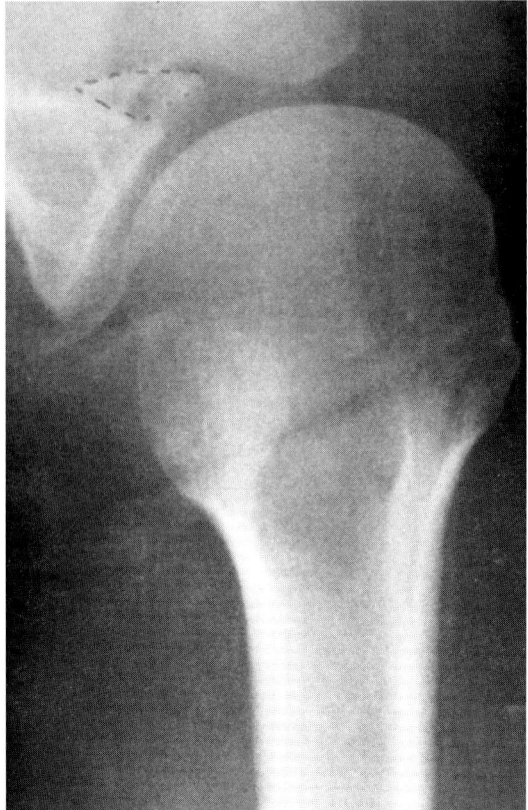

FIGURE 31
West Point axillary radiograph demonstrating an acute, anterior glenoid rim fracture with displacement.

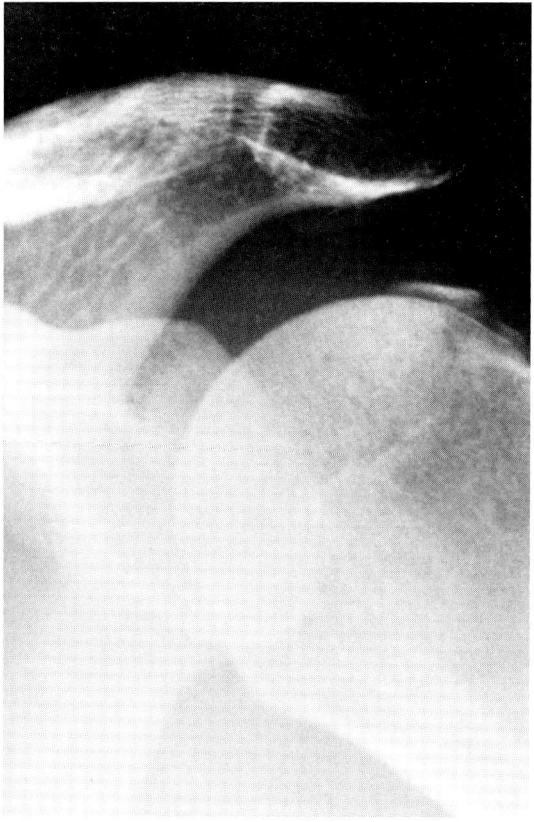

FIGURE 32
Routine anteroposterior radiograph with the humerus in internal rotation demonstrating a greater tuberosity fracture after an initial dislocation.

After the dislocation is fully evaluated, initial treatment consists of a closed reduction. In an emergency room setting, intravenous sedation using benzodiazepines and analgesics may be required. However, if the dislocation is seen acutely, it can occasionally be reduced without medication.

There are many different techniques to reduce a dislocated shoulder. Perhaps the simplest method is the Stimson method, in which 10 to 15 lb of weight are suspended from the wrist of the injured extremity with the patient prone.[2] This method is a gravity-assisted reduction and may require up to 15 minutes to achieve reduction (Fig. 33). The traction-countertraction technique described by Rockwood is also safe and efficient. With this method, an assistant pulls countertraction with a linen sheet circled about the torso to stabilize the chest and scapula. The surgeon pulls traction on the injured extremity distally to effect reduction (Fig. 34).[2]

An excellent technique that facilitates reduction and may preclude the use of intravenous sedation is the use of intra-articular lidocaine to achieve anesthesia. In this technique, 20 cc of 0.5% lidocaine is injected posteriorly into the shoulder joint and subacromial space. The injection should be placed 2 cm inferior and medial to the posterior lateral aspect of the acromion for the intra-articular component (15 cc). The needle can be redirected more superficially for the subacromial component (5 cc). This usually allows enough muscle relaxation to achieve a gentle reduction without an overly forceful manipulation. Digital pressure on the dislocated head under the coracoid often will help reduce the shoulder.

After reduction it is important to repeat and document the neurovascular examination.

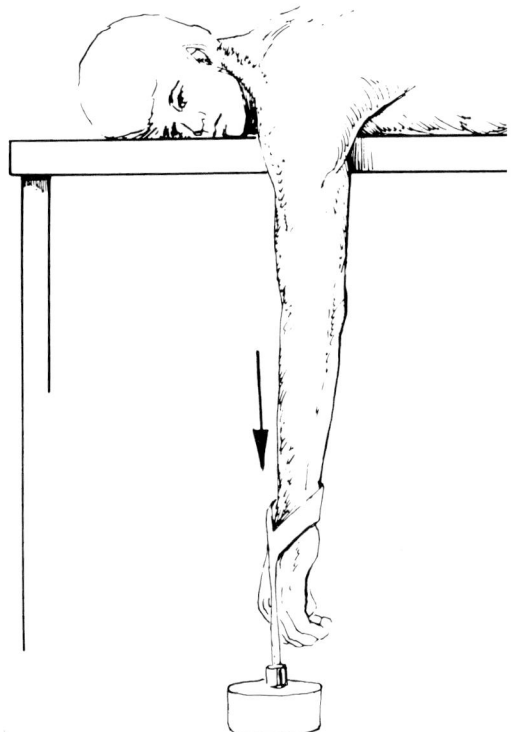

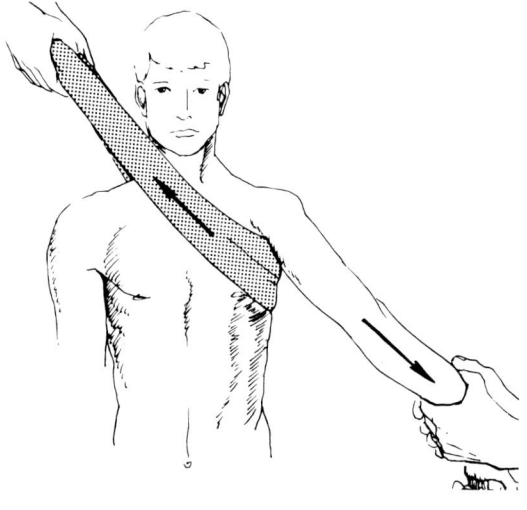

FIGURE 34

Traction–counter-traction method for reduction of an anterior dislocation of the shoulder. (Reproduced with permission from Warner JJP, Caborn DNM: Overview of shoulder instability. *Crit Rev Phys Rehab Med* 1992;4:145–190.)

NONSURGICAL TREATMENT

The vast majority of patients who sustain an acute, initial, traumatic anterior shoulder dislocation can be treated by a nonsurgical regimen that consists of a period of immobilization, supervised rehabilitation of shoulder girdle muscles, and a period of restriction from return to full activity. The purpose is to allow sufficient time for soft-tissue healing while minimizing recurrent instability, the main complication of shoulder dislocation.

Immobilization is somewhat controversial. Some authors have recommended no immobilization, while others advocate up to 6 weeks of complete immobilization. A sling and swathe or a commercial shoulder immobilizer can be used to limit abduction and external rotation while allowing healing of the capsule, labrum, and muscles. The immobilizer is used to support the arm and relieve pain and muscle spasm, usually for 2 to 3 weeks after acute pain and muscle spasm have subsided. Shoulder motion should be increased gradually.

A specific rehabilitation program should be started to strengthen the muscles of the shoulder and scapula. The dynamic stabilization function of the rotator cuff needs to be maximized to main-

FIGURE 33

Prone gravity-assisted reduction of an anterior dislocation as described by Stimson. (Reproduced with permission from Rockwood CA: Fractures and dislocations of the shoulder, in Rockwood CA, Green DP (eds): *Fractures in Adults,* ed 2. Philadelphia, PA, JB Lippincott, 1984, pp 722-805.)

Postreduction radiographs are also necessary to evaluate the adequacy of the reduction or to determine whether any further injury occurred during the maneuver. Furthermore, there should be a follow-up examination 7 to 10 days after injury, especially in patients older than 40 years of age. In these patients, a concomitant rotator cuff tear can occur, which may require further treatment.[6,7]

The initial evaluation of anterior instability should concentrate on the physical examination for other soft-tissue lesions involving the axillary nerve, axillary artery, and rotator cuff. Plain radiographs will confirm the direction of dislocation and diagnose other associated fractures of the greater tuberosity and glenoid fossa that may require treatment. After reduction, this evaluation must be repeated to rule out these other important soft-tissue and bony injuries.

tain stability.[8,9] The rehabilitation program should emphasize strengthening of the internal rotators, primarily the subscapularis, because this is an important stabilizer for anterior translation.[8-13] The supraspinatus, infraspinatus, and teres minor are especially important in overhead sports and they affect translation.[8] These muscles can be strengthened in a rehabilitation program that uses pulleys, rubber tubing, or progressive resistance rubber bands.[10,12] The serratus anterior, trapezius, and levator scapulae are critical scapular stabilizers that provide optimal positioning of the glenoid fossa during shoulder abduction and external rotation and maximize glenohumeral stability.[8,12] These muscles can be strengthened by push-ups and the push-ups plus exercise. Recently, Itoi and associates[11] demonstrated in vitro the stabilizing effect of the biceps tendon. In a cadaveric study, both the short and long heads of the biceps tendon resisted anterior translation.[11] The authors recommend rehabilitation programs that include strengthening the biceps tendon. As pain decreases and strength increases, free weights and more sophisticated weight machines can be used to achieve optimum neuromuscular control.

In a classic report, Rowe and Sakellarides[14] described the results of nonsurgical treatment in 524 primary dislocations. The recurrence rate was 94% in patients between 11 and 20 years of age, 74% in patients 20 to 40 years of age, and 14% in those older than 40 years. Rowe recommended immobilization for 3 weeks, but found a reduction in recurrence of only 10% to 15%. In an independent study, McLaughlin documented a recurrence rate of 95% in 181 patients younger than 20 years of age.[15,16] Kiviluoto and associates[17] reported that in the first year after the primary dislocation, the rate of recurrence was 56% in patients younger than 20 and 36% in all patients younger than 30 years old. Immobilization for 3 weeks decreased the recurrence rate. Henry and Genung[18] described a recurrence rate of 88% in a very athletic population with an average age of 19 years. Immobilization was not found to have any beneficial effect in diminishing recurrence. The authors believe that primary surgical repair should be considered in certain conditions.

Simonet and Cofield[19] demonstrated that recurrence rates may not be quite as high as previously reported. In 116 patients studied, the overall recurrence rate was 33%. For patients younger than 20 years old, the recurrence rate was still 66%; for those between 20 and 40 years of age, the rate was 40%. However, the recurrence rate in "athletes" younger than 30 years of age was 82%. Symptomatic instability other than dislocation (ie, subluxation) was significant in another 25% of the patients. This study was important because follow-up was excellent and both age *and* athletic activity were demonstrated to be important factors for recurrence. Patients who were restricted from return to full activity for at least 6 weeks did better than those who were allowed earlier return.

In a study of 63 hockey players, Hovelius[20] reported the recurrence rate in players younger than 20 years of age to be 90%; in those 20 to 25 years of age, the rate was 65%; and in patients older than 25 years of age, the rate was 50%.[20] The largest study of primary dislocations involved 257 patients followed for at least 10 years.[21] The overall recurrence rate for dislocation was 48%, 23% required surgery, and dislocation arthropathy was reported in 20%. Hovelius[22,23] reported that immobilization, type of trauma, bilateral involvement, family history, and athletic activity did not affect recurrence. However, his experience with Swedish hockey players—a young, high-demand group—demonstrated a much higher incidence of recurrence and need for surgery than reported in the 10-year report as a whole.

These six reports suggest a minimum recurrence rate of 56% after the initial dislocation with several reports as high as 95% in patients younger than 20 years of age.

Two reports add significant controversy to the expected results of nonsurgical treatment for acute dislocation. Yoneda and associates[24] reported a 17% recurrence rate in 104 patients with an average follow-up of 13 years. These patients averaged 21.5 years of age and were immobilized for 5 weeks followed by 6 weeks of graduated exercise. Aronen and Regan[13] reported a 25% recurrence in 20 US Naval Academy midshipmen who were immobilized for 3 weeks, followed by a well-supervised rehabilitation program. The results of these two investigations suggest that immobilization combined with rehabilitation may impact on recurrence rates. However, neither of these studies had a control group or similar cohort. In addition, the effects of both immobilization and rehabilitation have been at best inconsistent in this age group. Other studies of young athletes have reported recurrence rates of 82% to 95%.

It is difficult to summarize and make firm recommendations from the results of these reports of nonsurgical treatment. The primary prognostic factor for recurrence is age. Patients younger than 20 years of age have the highest recurrence rates (up to 95%); patients between 21 and 30 years, from 37% to 70%; and those aged 30 to 40 years, 12% to 40%. After the age of 40, recurrence rates are low.

It would appear that nonsurgical treatment of the initial anterior dislocation should include a period of immobilization. This should allow for soft-tissue healing. The results of previous reports suggest there *may* be some benefit from up to 3 weeks immobilization in young patients. In general, the older the patient, the shorter the immobilization period so as to avoid stiffness. Furthermore, a specific rehabilitation program combined with a delay in return to full activity until full rehabilitation of the internal rotators also appears justified.

However, an athlete younger than 22 years of age has the greatest risk for recurrence despite nonsurgical treatment. At the US Military Academy, a unique opportunity exists to evaluate the natural history and management of initial anterior dislocations. This population of young athletes with high risk are unwilling to modify their activity. The failure of nonsurgical treatment to decrease recurrences at this institution has stimulated several studies evaluating acute arthroscopic repair.

SURGICAL TREATMENT

The cadets at the US Military Academy represent a uniform population of young athletes with an age range of 17 to 24 years. In addition to intercollegiate, intramural, and club sports participation, there are physical education requirements for graduation that include boxing, wrestling, rugby, and obstacle courses. Yearly military training includes hand-to-hand combat, pugil sticks, and parachute training. Within this environment, acute shoulder instability is a frequent clinical problem.

Wheeler and associates[25] reported on 35 of 38 cadets (average age, 19.5 years) who developed recurrent instability with nonsurgical treatment after the initial dislocation. These patients were immobilized for 3 weeks, underwent supervised rehabilitation, and then returned to full activity

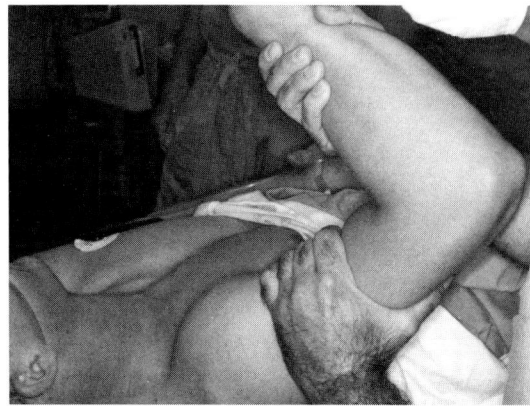

FIGURE 35
Load and shift laxity examination of the glenohumeral joint in the plane of the scapula and with 90° of abduction. The examiner's left hand can be used to direct an anterior, inferior, or posterior force while the humeral head is centered within the glenoid fossa. The amount of translation is graded as 0, 1+, 2+, or 3+.

3 months after injury. During this time, nine patients consented to arthroscopic treatment. Two patients (22%) developed recurrence. Although the surgical group was small, results suggested that acute arthroscopic repair may significantly improve the results.

Recently, the results of a second prospective study evaluating nonsurgical and arthroscopic treatment for the initial dislocation were reported.[5] Each patient required a manual reduction as initial treatment. In the nonsurgical group, patients were immobilized for 4 weeks, underwent supervised rehabilitation, and returned to full activity at 4 months. Twelve of 15 cadets (average age, 19.6) sustained recurrences with seven (47%) requiring subsequent open Bankart repair. The surgical group underwent arthroscopic transglenoid suture repair within 10 days of injury and followed the same protocol as the nonsurgical group.[26] By contrast, three of 21 patients treated arthroscopically developed recurrences at an average follow-up of 32 months. One patient required an open Bankart repair.

Together, these two studies included the first 30 patients at the US Military Academy who were treated with arthroscopic repair after the initial anterior dislocation. These initial studies were important for several reasons. In each case, examination under anesthesia showed increased anterior translation with the modified load and shift test (Fig. 35) (RF Warren, personal communication).

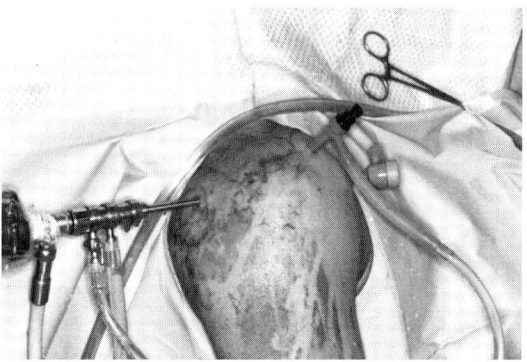

FIGURE 36
Right shoulder arthroscopy in the sitting position demonstrating the traditional posterior viewing portal, an anterior superior portal, and an anterior inferior portal.

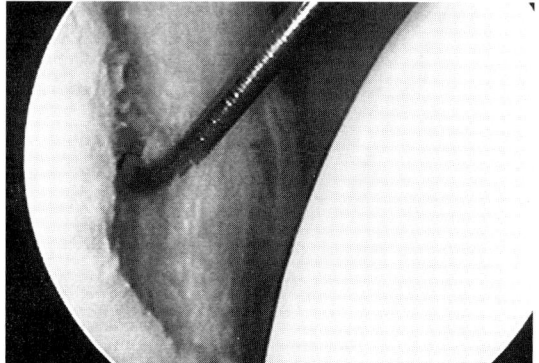

FIGURE 37
Arthroscopic view of an acute, initial anterior dislocation in a right shoulder. Note the robust appearing labrum and tissue after the initial dislocation.

OUTLINE 2 CLINICAL AND ARTHROSCOPIC FINDINGS OF INITIAL, ANTERIOR DISLOCATION*

Age[†]	19.6
Males	59
Females	6
Sport of injury	
Collision	28
Limited contact	26
Noncontact	2
Bony Bankart on West Point view	12
Arthroscopic findings	
Hemarthrosis	65
Bankart lesion	63
Hill-Sachs lesion	53
SLAP lesion	6
Humeral detachment of inferior glenohumeral ligament	1
Capsular tear	1

*N = 65
[†]Range = 17 to 24 years

The arthroscopic pathology was also well documented. A hemarthrosis and an avulsion of the capsule and labrum from the anterior glenoid (Perthes; Bankart lesion) was observed in each case. These arthroscopic findings are similar to those reported previously. Baker and associates[27] reported that either partial or complete capsulo-labral disruption occurred in 39 of 45 patients (87%) who underwent arthroscopic examination after an initial dislocation that required a reduction. They described three injury patterns observed acutely: six of 45 patients had a capsular injury and these patients had a stable examination under anesthesia; 11 shoulders had subluxation on examination that had a partial labral detachment; 28 shoulders were dislocatable and had a complete labral detachment. Norlin[28] recently reported a 100% incidence of a Bankart lesion in 24 patients who were evaluated with arthroscopy after a first-time dislocation. It is interesting to note that Thomas and Matsen[29] reported a 97% incidence of avulsion of the IGHL in their study of recurrent, *traumatic,* anterior instability of the shoulder. The point of emphasis is that in *traumatic* instability, the pathologic findings of avulsion of the IGHL complex is observed with high frequency. Finally, arthroscopic repair of these first 24 patients appeared to significantly reduce the rate of recurrent instability compared to nonsurgical treatment. Although the follow-up is still early, the results have been superior to nonsurgical treatment.

Recently, the sitting position and interscalene anesthesia have been used for arthroscopy (Fig. 36)[30] and the repair technique has been changed from the transglenoid suture repair to one utilizing a bioabsorbable tack.[31-33] This avoids drilling through the scapula with its risk of suprascapular nerve injury. The tack allows direct repair to bone without tying suture over the posterior soft tissues. This technique has been used in an additional 35 cadets to treat a traumatic anterior initial dislocation. The arthroscopic findings have been similar in this group. All patients had a hemarthrosis and 33 of 35 had a Bankart lesion. The typical pathology visualized shows tissue of excellent quality with the capsulolabral complex of the IGHL detached from the glenoid and scapular neck (Fig. 37). With the exception of one case, no *gross* capsular damage has been observed. There was one *lateral* detachment of the IGHL from the neck of the proximal humerus.[34] The Hill-Sachs lesion has been observed in approximately 87% of the cases. There have been four superior labral anterior-to-posterior (SLAP) lesions, of which two required stabilization with an additional 6-mm tack.[35,36] At an average follow-up of 21 months, three recurrences have been reported. The average Rowe score was 92 points (range, 50 to 100 points). Two patients sustained recurrent dislocation with collision sports. One patient developed recurrent subluxation after reinjury on an obstacle course 10 months after repair. No other complications related to this treatment were reported.

Therefore, since 1986, 120 patients at the US Military Academy have been treated for an initial traumatic anterior shoulder dislocation. The average age has been approximately 20 years. In each case, a manual reduction was required. Fifty-five patients were treated nonsurgically and recurrent symptomatic instability developed in 47 (85%). Arthroscopic evaluation and treatment using three different arthroscopic techniques was performed in 65 patients. A summary of these arthroscopic findings is provided in Outline 2. All patients returned to preinjury activity level. Eight patients (12%) developed recurrent instability.

Based on the experience with this technique, it is thought that the young athlete (younger than 24 years of age), who historically is at risk for recurrence after the initial dislocation, is a candidate for acute repair. This treatment has been reserved for the dislocation that requires reduction and in patients without any preceding shoulder problem. Although the results of arthroscopic stabilization in chronic instability have been less favorable to date than results of open techniques, the acute, initial dislocation is a different circumstance.[37-39] After an acute, initial dislocation, a hemarthrosis is consistently present and the avulsed capsulolabral complex of the inferior glenohumeral ligament is in the best condition for repair. There is no labral degeneration or marked capsular attenuation, as is frequently observed in chronic instability. These unique pathologic conditions may be optimal for an arthroscopic stabilization technique.

There are other indications for surgery in the acute setting. Surgery is necessary for reduction in patients who sustain an associated displaced greater tuberosity fracture. Displaced fractures (more than 1 cm) will compromise rotator cuff function and can lead to subacromial impingement.[40] Frequently, CT is necessary to determine accurately the amount of displacement.[41]

Anterior dislocations in middle-aged patients frequently have an associated rotator cuff tear that may require surgical repair, especially in active patients. The incidence of this complication increases with age. In patients older than 40 years, the incidence exceeds 30%.[4,6]

In rare instances, an irreducible dislocation may be encountered. Case reports of soft-tissue interposition involving the rotator cuff, capsule, or biceps tendon been described, necessitating open reduction.[2]

REFERENCES

1. Blom S, Dahlback LO: Nerve injuries in dislocations of the shoulder joint and fractures of the neck of the humerus: A clinical and electromyographical study. *Acta Chir Scand* 1970;136:461-466.

2. Neer CS II, Rockwood CA Jr: Fractures and dislocations of the shoulder, in Rockwood CA Jr, Green DP (eds): *Fractures in Adults,* ed 2. Philadelphia, PA, JB Lippincott, 1984, vol 1, pp 675-985.

3. Neer CS II: Anatomy of shoulder reconstruction, in Neer CS II (ed): *Shoulder Reconstruction.* Philadelphia, PA, WB Saunders, 1990, pp 1 39.

4. Rokous JR, Feagin JA, Abbott HG: Modified axillary roentgenogram: A useful adjunct in the diagnosis of recurrent instability of the shoulder. *Clin Orthop* 1972;82:84-86.

5. Arciero RA, Wheeler JH, Ryan JB, et al: Arthroscopic Bankart repair versus non-operative treatment for acute, initial anterior shoulder dislocations. *Am J Sports Med* 1994;22:589-594.

6. Tijmes J, Loyd HM, Tullos HS: Arthrography in acute shoulder dislocations. *South Med J* 1979;72:564-567.

7. Ribbans WJ, Mitchell R, Taylor GJ: Computerised arthrotomography of primary anterior dislocation of the shoulder. *J Bone Joint Surg* 1990:72B:181-185.

8. Glousman R, Jobe F, Tibone JD, et al: Dynamic electromyographic analysis of the throwing shoulder with glenohumeral instability. *J Bone Joint Surg* 1988;70A:220-226.

9. Warner JJ, Micheli LJ, Arslanian LE, et al: Patterns of flexibility, laxity, and strength in normal shoulders and shoulders with instability and impingement. *Am J Sports Med* 1990;18:366-375.

10. Burkhead WZ Jr, Rockwood CA Jr: Treatment of instability of the shoulder with an exercise program. *J Bone Joint Surg* 1992;74A:890-896.

11. Itoi E, Kuechle DK, Newman SR, et al: Stabilizing function of the biceps in stable and unstable shoulders. *J Bone Joint Surg* 1993;75B:546-550.

12. Jobe FW, Moynes DR, Brewster CE: Rehabilitation of shoulder joint instabilities. *Orthop Clin North Am* 1987;18:473-482.

13. Aronen JG, Regan K: Decreasing the incidence of recurrence of first time anterior shoulder dislocations with rehabilitation. *Am J Sports Med* 1984;12:283-291.

14. Rowe CR, Sakellarides HT: Factors related to recurrences of anterior dislocations of the shoulder. *Clin Orthop* 1961;20:40-48.

15. McLaughlin HL, Cavallaro WU: Primary anterior dislocation of the shoulder. *Am J Surg* 1950;80:615-621.

16. McLaughlin HL, MacLellan DI: Recurrent anterior dislocation of the shoulder: II. A comparative study. *J Trauma* 1967;7:191-201.

17. Kiviluoto O, Pasila M, Jaroma H, et al: Immobilization after primary dislocation of the shoulder. *Acta Orthop Scand* 1980;51:915-919.

18. Henry JH, Genung JA: Natural history of glenohumeral dislocation: Revisited. *Am J Sports Med* 1982;10:135-137.

19. Simonet WT, Cofield RH: Prognosis in anterior shoulder dislocation. *Am J Sports Med* 1984;12:19-24.

20. Hovelius L: Shoulder dislocation in Swedish ice hockey players. *Am J Sports Med* 1978;6:373-377.

21. Hovelius L, Malmqvist B, Augustini BG, et al: Abstract: Ten year prognosis of primary anterior dislocation of the shoulder in the young, in *Programs and Abstracts of the 10th Open Meeting of the American Shoulder and Elbow Surgeons.* New Orleans, LA, 1994, p 17.

22. Hovelius L, Eriksson K, Fredin H, et al: Recurrences after initial dislocation of the shoulder: Results of a prospective study of treatment. *J Bone Joint Surg* 1983;65A:343-349.

23. Hovelius L: Anterior dislocation of the shoulder in teenagers and young adults. *J Bone Joint Surg* 1987;69A:393-399.

24. Yoneda B, Welsh RP, MacIntosh DL: Conservative treatment of shoulder dislocation in young males. *J Bone Joint Surg* 1982;64B:254-255.

25. Wheeler JH, Ryan JB, Arciero RA, et al: Arthroscopic versus nonoperative treatment of acute shoulder dislocations in young athletes. *Arthroscopy* 1989;5:213-217.

26. Morgan CD, Bodenstab AB: Arthroscopic Bankart suture repair: Technique and early results. *Arthroscopy* 1987;3:111-122.

27. Baker CL, Uribe JW, Whitman C: Arthroscopic evaluation of acute initial anterior shoulder dislocations. *Am J Sports Med* 1990;18:25-28.

28. Norlin R: Intraarticular pathology in acute, first-time anterior shoulder dislocation: An arthroscopic study. *Arthroscopy* 1993;9:546-549.

29. Thomas SC, Matsen FA III: An approach to the repair of avulsion of the glenohumeral ligaments in the management of traumatic anterior glenohumeral instability. *J Bone Joint Surg* 1989;71A:506-513.

30. Skyhar MJ, Altchek DW, Warren RF, et al: Shoulder Arthroscopy with the patient in the beach-chair position. *Arthroscopy* 1988;4:256-259.

31. Altchek DW: Arthroscopic shoulder stabilization using a bioabsorbable fixation device. *Sports Med Arthroscopy Rev* 1993;1:266-271.

32. Pagnani MJ, Warren RF: Arthroscopic shoulder stabilization. *Op Tech Sports Med* 1993;1:276-284.

33. Warner JJP, Warren RF: Arthroscopic Bankart repair using a cannulated, absorbable fixation device. *Op Tech Orthop* 1991;1:192-198.

34. Bach BR, Warren RF, Fronek J: Disruption of the lateral capsule of the shoulder: A cause of recurrent dislocation. *J Bone Joint Surg* 1988;70B:274-276.

35. Snyder SJ, Karzel RP, Del Pizzo W, et al: SLAP lesions of the shoulder. *Arthroscopy* 1990;6:274-279.

36. Warner JJ, Kann S, Marks P: Arthroscopic repair of combined Bankart and superior labral detachment anterior and posterior lesions: Technique and preliminary results. *Arthroscopy* 1994;10:383-391.

37. Coughlin L, Rubinovich M, Johansson J, et al: Arthroscopic staple capsulorrhaphy for anterior shoulder instability. *Am J Sports Med* 1992;20:253-256.

38. Hawkins RB: Arthroscopic stapling repair for shoulder instability: A retrospective study of 50 cases. *Arthroscopy* 1989;5:122-128.

39. Matthews LS, Vetter WL, Oweida SJ, et al: Arthroscopic staple capsulorrhaphy for recurrent anterior shoulder instability. *Arthroscopy* 1988;4:106-111.

40. Neer CS II: Displaced proximal humeral fractures: Part I. Classification and evaluation. *J Bone Joint Surg* 1970;52A:1077-1089.

41. Norris TR, Bigliani LU: Complications following the modified Bristow procedure for shoulder instability. *Orthop Trans* 1987;11:232-233.

RECURRENT ANTERIOR INSTABILITY: ARTHROSCOPIC REPAIR

JON J.P. WARNER, MD

NONSURGICAL TREATMENT

Nonsurgical treatment of recurrent anterior shoulder instability involves activity modification and a specific rotator cuff and scapular stabilizer strengthening program. Athletes injured during the athletic season often defer surgery until after the season. Restrictive devices to limit the amount of abduction and external rotation are helpful in such patients.[1] Several leather, canvas, and plastic harnesses or braces are commercially available to restrain the affected shoulder girdle. Although no randomized prospective studies have evaluated these devices, because they limit motion they have been helpful in diminishing instability events.

The effects of a specific exercise program to treat recurrent shoulder instability depends on the type of instability pattern. Burkhead and Rockwood[2] examined the results of a specific exercise program to treat shoulder instability and reported that in patients with atraumatic and often multidirectional instability 53 of 66 shoulders (80%) were successfully treated with an exercise program. In contrast, only 12 of 74 shoulders (16%) with traumatic instability were successfully treated with the exercise program.

ARTHROSCOPIC BANKART REPAIR

RATIONALE

Historically, traumatic, recurrent anterior shoulder instability has been well managed by open Bankart repair techniques.[3] Nevertheless, over the past 2 decades shoulder arthroscopy has evolved from a diagnostic application into a treatment approach. This interest in arthroscopic repair of shoulder instability has been based on perceived disadvantages of open repair techniques. Some of these concerns include loss of motion (especially external rotation), poor cosmesis of a surgical

incision, postoperative pain and surgical morbidity, and the technical difficulties encountered in open Bankart repair. Arthroscopic repair techniques have been described as offering the advantages of faster surgery with less surgical morbidity, reduced postoperative pain, selective anatomic repair of the Bankart lesion without dissection through adjacent normal tissues, recovery of more normal range of motion, and improved speed and ease for the surgeon.[4-6] Some of these theoretical advantages have occurred in the clinical experience of some shoulder arthroscopists; however, the recurrence rate of glenohumeral instability following arthroscopic repair remains higher than for open procedures and complications have occurred.

Historical Overview The most popular repair techniques have been staple fixation[7-18] (Table 2) and transosseous suture repair[19-37] (Table 3). The staple repair technique pioneered by Johnson[7] formed the basis for subsequent arthroscopic approaches. His initial experience was marked by a failure rate of about 20%, which was largely attributed to permitting patients motion in the early postoperative period. When patients were immobilized for 4 weeks postoperatively, this failure rate decreased by half. Unfortunately, the experience of other surgeons has been that staple fixation is fraught with a variety of complications, including breakage and migration of the implants as well as articular injury (Table 2 and Fig. 38).[9,13,15,16,37,38]

For these reasons, Caspari and Savoie,[21] Morgan,[28,29] and others[19,20,22-27,30-36] (Table 3) developed arthroscopic suture repair techniques. These techniques were based on the transosseous open Bankart repair procedure developed by Reider and Inglis.[39] After first decorticating the anterior glenoid rim, the surgeon places sutures through an anterior cannula into the IGHL and labrum and drills several long metal pins through the juxta-articular anterior scapula so that they exit

TABLE 2

ARTHROSCOPIC BANKART REPAIR WITH STAPLE TECHNIQUE

Series	Number of Patients	Mean Follow-up (months)	Recurrence (%)	Comments
Small (1986)*	562	—	—	Loose staples (14)
Matthews (1988)	25	36	20	Staple impingement (1)
Wiley (1988)	10	6 to 24	17	Removable rivet
Hawkins (1989)	50	39	16	Loose staples (4)
Wheeler (1989)	9	more than 17	16	
Gross (1989)	12	45	33	Staple impingement (1)
Burger (1990)	52	25	13	Loose staples (3)
Coughlin (1992)	47	48	25	Painful staples (3)
Lane (1993)	54	39	33	Loose staples (11%)
Wilson (1993)	101	16.3	27	
Johnson (1993)	Series 1, 77	24	21	More than 3 weeks in sling
	Series 2, 124	36	14	Pain (47%)
Rao (1994)	22	28	26	Pain (60%)

*Review article

TABLE 3

ARTHROSCOPIC BANKART REPAIR WITH SUTURE TECHNIQUE [*]

Series	Number of Patients	Mean Follow-up (months)	Recurrence (%)
Morgan (1987)	25	17	—
Wolin (1990)	45	>24	27
Weber (1990)	23	27	17
Rose (1990)	50	>24	4
Caspari (1991)	49	24-72	4
Morgan (1991)	55	49	4
(1991)	120	12-36	5.8
(1991)	42	—	16.6
Landsiedl (1992)	65	35	11
Benedetto (1992)	31	24	0
Duncan (1993)	10	12-36	0
Neviaser (1993)	26	> 24	4
Goldberg (1993)	38	"Preliminary"	10
Grana (1993)	27	36	45
Geiger (1993)	16	23	44
Foster (1994)	75	12-84	8
Arciero (1994)	21	32	14
Walch (1994)	59	2 to 6 years	40
Pagnani (1994)	37	4 to 10 years	19

* Arthroscopic capsular shift for multidirectional instability.

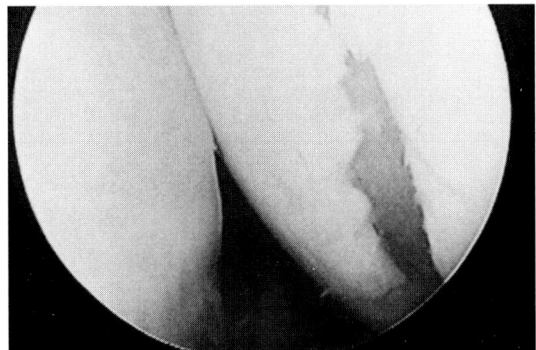

FIGURE 38
Arthroscopic Bankart repair with staple fixation placed too high on the glenoid rim and in an intra-articular position.

through the infraspinatus fossa. The sutures are then passed through the hole in the end of each pin and pulled through the drill holes so that they can be tied over the infraspinatus muscle through a separate small posterior incision (Fig. 39).

Although initial experience of expert arthroscopists[21,29] has been favorable, with failure rates less than 8%, others have had unacceptably high recurrence rates in both short- and long-term follow-up (Table 3). Two recent reports by experienced arthroscopic shoulder surgeons[31,36] have documented a failure rate of over 40% at a minimum 3-year follow-up. There are several explanations for this high failure rate. First, the technique is difficult and it may not always be possible to adequately place sutures into the IGHL so that it is securely snugged up to the anterior-inferior glenoid. Second, tying the sutures over the infraspinatus muscle posteriorly may not allow secure compression of the IGHL and labrum against the anterior-inferior glenoid because there may be some elastic "give" of the soft tissues that permits the Bankart repair to "gap." Third, absorbable and nonabsorbable monofilament suture material is often used because of its ease of passage through the suture passer and soft tissues; this material has been shown to be suboptimal for soft tissue to bone repair because of its elastic characteristics.[40] Recent development of suture passers that allow the use of braided, nonabsorbable material will eliminate this concern. Fourth, there is a risk of iatrogenic injury to neurovascular structures from errant pin placement.[37,38] The fifth, and probably the most common reason that this technique fails, is poor patient selection. Patients with ligamentous laxity

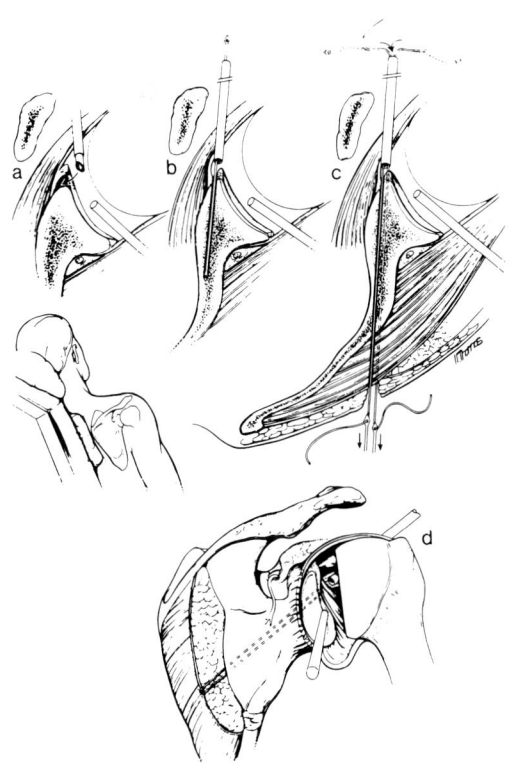

FIGURE 39
Arthroscopic trans-scapular suture repair technique. **a,** Visualization of the Bankart lesion. **b,** Drilling of the beath pin across the scapula. **c,** Passage of the beath pin and suture through an accessory posterior incision in the infraspinatus. **d,** Sutures are tied over the infraspinatus muscle repairing the Bankart lesion anteriorly. (Reproduced with permission from Pagnani MJ, Galinat BJ, Warren RF: Glenohumeral instability, in DeLee JC, Drez D Jr (eds): *Orthopaedic Sports Medicine: Principles and Practice.* Philadelphia, PA, WB Saunders, 1994, p 604.)

or intraligamentous injury (Fig. 40) may not be appropriate candidates for an arthroscopic approach. There appears to be a higher recurrence rate in contact and collision sport athletes.[21,35,41]

Technique In order to avoid some of the technical problems and complications associated with arthroscopic staple and suture repair methods, absorbable, cannulated fixation devices have been developed (Fig. 41).[6,41-44] Several devices have been proposed but the one most commonly used is composed of polyglyconate polymer that loses its

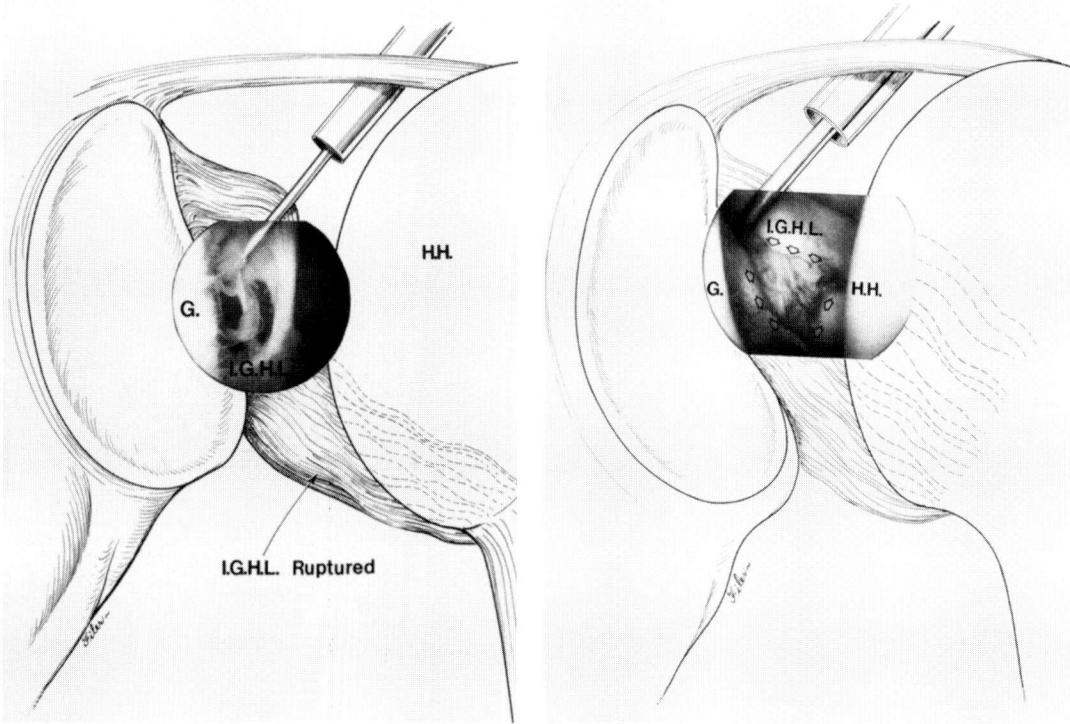

FIGURE 40
Rupture of the inferior glenohumeral ligament (IGHL) with anterior dislocation. **Left,** Patient with chronic recurrent dislocations. **Right,** Patient with an acute anterior dislocation. The inferior glenohumeral ligament (IGHL), glenoid (G), and humeral head (HH) are labelled for orientation.

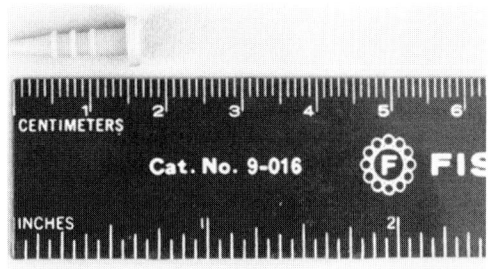

FIGURE 41
The Suretac® device (see text).

strength as it resorbs. It basically acts as a temporary compressive fixation for soft-tissue repair to bone over a 4-week period.[41-44] This offers the advantages of direct repair of the capsulolabral separation (Bankart lesion) with tissue compression underneath a 6- or 8-mm head. In addition, there

are no concerns about articular injury from impingement of the implant and there is no need for an accessory posterior incision, as would be required with some of the suture repair techniques.

Patients are selected for arthroscopic repair based on a history of traumatic, recurrent, unidirectional anterior shoulder subluxation or dislocation. Specifically excluded are patients with a history of atraumatic instability, voluntary instability, and evidence of marked laxity of the glenohumeral joint in multiple planes. This selection process is described in further detail in the subsequent section of the text.

Interscalene regional anesthesia is preferred for this procedure because it appears to reduce complications such as nausea, fatigue, and morbidity of general anesthesia, allowing most patients to go home on the day of surgery.

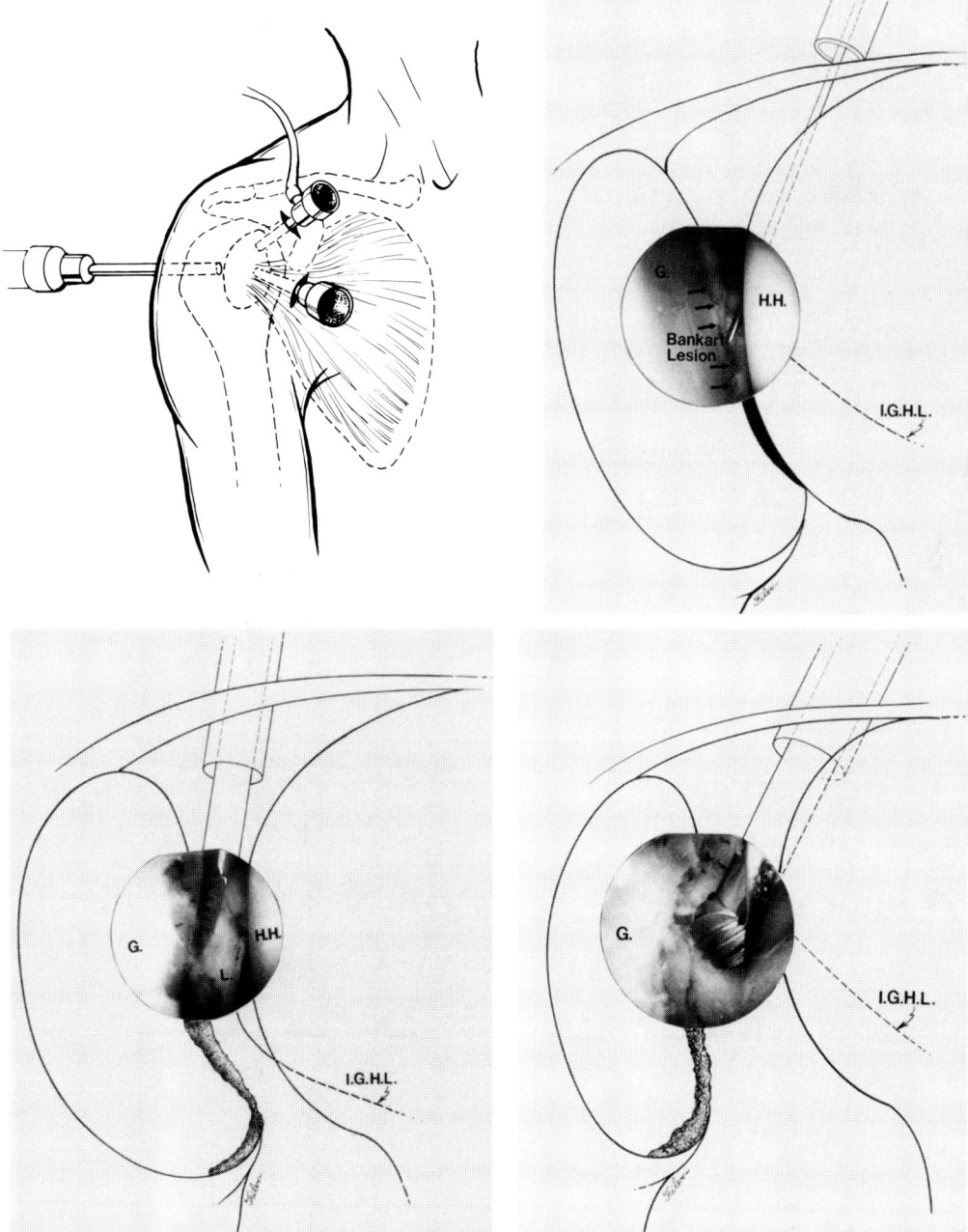

FIGURE 42

Top left, Portals for arthroscopic Bankart repair (see text). **Top right,** A Bankart lesion as seen through the posterior portal with a probe placed through the anterior-superior portal. The inferior glenohumeral ligament (IGHL) and humeral head (HH) are labelled. **Bottom left,** Mobilization of the labrum (L) and inferior glenohumeral ligament (IGHL) off the juxta-articular anterior and inferior scapular rim. The glenoid (G) and humeral head (HH) are labelled for orientation. **Bottom right,** An arthroscopic burr is used to decorticate the anterior-inferior scapular neck prior to Bankart repair. (Reproduced with permission from Warner JJP, Miller MD, Marks PH, et al: Arthroscopic Bankart repair with the Suretac® device: Part 1. Clinical observations. *Arthroscopy* 1995;11:2-13.)

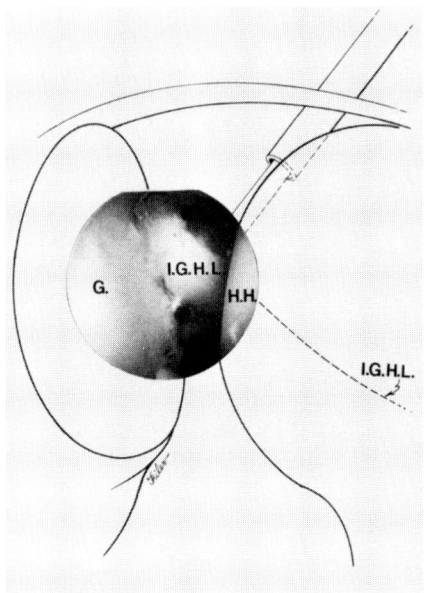
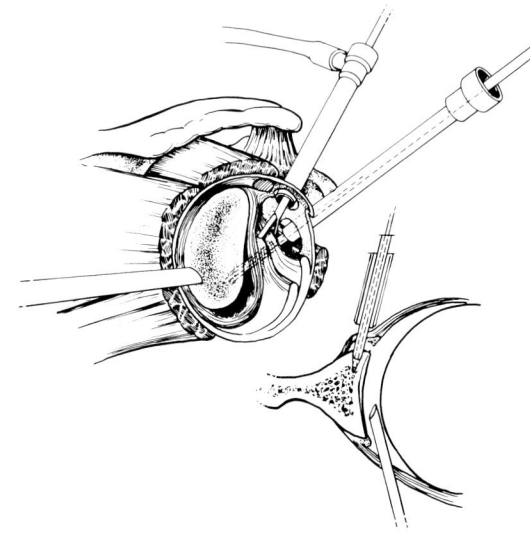

FIGURE 43

Left, Arthroscopic view through the posterior portal of the drill-guidewire through the inferior glenohumeral ligament (IGHL) at the 4 to 5 o'clock position. (Reproduced with permission from Warner JJP, Miller MD, Marks PH, et al: Arthroscopic Bankart repair with the Suretac® device: Part 1. Clinical observations. *Arthroscopy* 1995;11:2-13.) **Right,** Diagram showing proper placement of the drill-guidewire for insertion of the first Suretac. (Reproduced with permission from Warner JJP, Warren RF: Arthroscopic Bankart repair with an absorbable, cannulated fixation device. *Oper Tech Orthop* 1991;1:192-198.)

Although many surgeons perform shoulder arthroscopy with the patient in a lateral decubitus position, the upright "beach-chair" position is advantageous for several reasons (Fig. 42).[6,42] First, it allows free shoulder rotation that permits assessment of the quality and character of the glenohumeral ligaments. An attempt is made to define the magnitude and location of capsuloligamentous injury as well as the development or robustness of the glenohumeral ligaments. Individuals with thick, robust-appearing glenohumeral ligaments and a discrete Bankart lesion are better suited for arthroscopic repair than those with evidence of intracapsular injury or lax, patulous capsuloligamentous structures (Fig. 40). Specific attention is directed to the IGHL, which is probed and grasped to determine if it is lax or has been injured.

Second, when the patient is in a seated position the shoulder remains in adduction and this allows the subscapularis to fall inferiorly. This permits placement of the anteroinferior portal low enough so that the first bioabsorbable tack can be inserted at the anterior-inferior glenoid rim. Third, there is the potential for neurologic injury to the brachial plexus from the traction device. Fourth, conversion to an open approach is easy, when necessary, because the patient is already in a sitting position.

Surgical portal placement (Fig. 42) is the first important technical step. An anterior-superior portal is placed percutaneously so that the arthroscopic cannula enters the joint just underneath the biceps tendon. This portal allows the glenohumeral ligaments to be probed as well as the Bankart lesion to be prepared for the repair. An anterior-inferior portal is the principal portal used for instrumentation and tack insertion. It is important to place this cannula as low as possible into the joint so that the first tack can be inserted through the IGHL at the anterior-inferior rim of the glenoid (between the 4 and 5 o'clock positions for a right glenoid). A spinal needle is placed into the joint from a position 1 cm inferior and lateral to the coracoid process so that it enters the joint just over the subscapularis tendon. The orientation of the needle is noted and then the needle is removed and replaced with the instrumentation cannula. The juxta-articular scapular neck is prepared for Bankart repair and

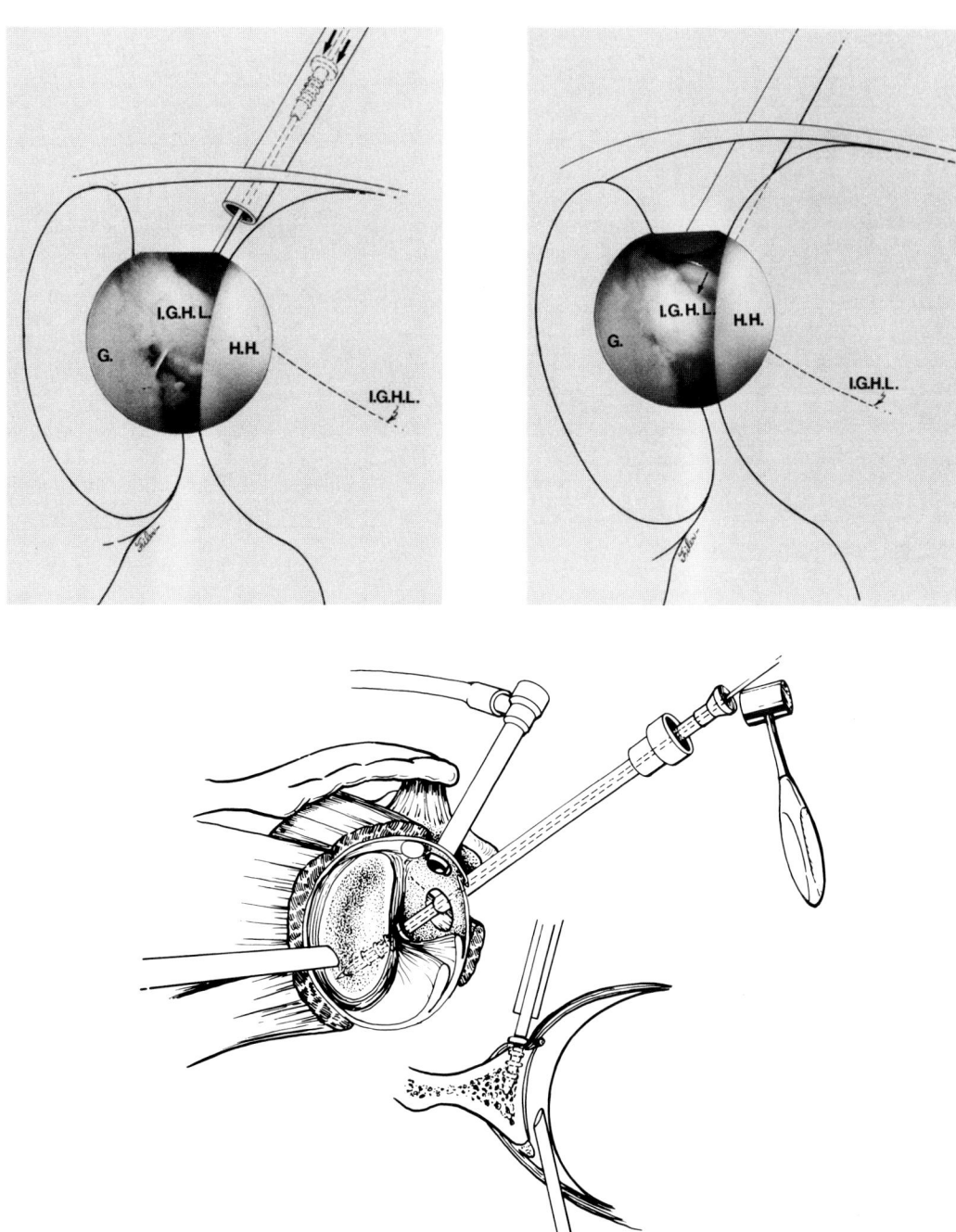

FIGURE 44

Procedure in FIGURE 43, continued. **Top left,** Insertion of the Suretac over the guidewire. **Top right,** Compression of the inferior glenohumeral ligament by the Suretac® device. (Reproduced with permission from Warner JJP, Miller MD, Marks PH, et al: Arthroscopic Bankart repair with the Suretac® device: Part 1. Clinical observations. *Arthroscopy* 1995;11:2-13.)
Bottom, Diagram of Suretac® insertion. (Reproduced with permission from Warner JJP, Miller MD, Marks PH: Arthroscopic Bankart repair with the Suretac® device: Part 2. Experimental observations. *Arthroscopy* 1995;11:14-20.)

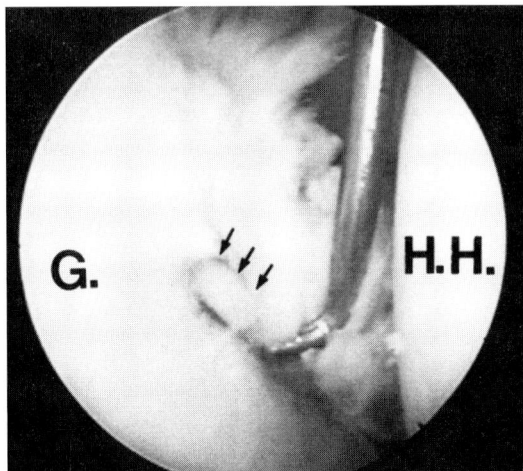

FIGURE 45
The Suretac has "buttonholed" (arrows) through the inferior glenohumeral ligament. The glenoid (G) and humeral head (HH) are labelled for orientation.

mobilization of the IGHL. An electrocautery device is used to enlarge the Bankart lesion by extending it inferiorly to the 6 o'clock position on the glenoid rim as well as subperiostially, dissecting along the scapula anteriorly and inferiorly (Fig. 42). A sharp rasp can be used to assist in this step. It is important to mobilize the IGHL in this manner so that it can be shifted superiorly and medially with the repair (Fig. 42).

The juxta-articular scapular neck is then abraded with an arthroscopic burr. It is important to take special care to place the burr through the anterior-inferior portal as well as the anterior-superior portal so that both the inferior rim and anterior rim are prepared (Fig. 42). This step ensures that there is soft tissue to bone healing and that a trough is created that prevents the drill from slipping either medially or laterally during the repair.

When a Bankart lesion occurs, the IGHL is detached in an anterior and inferior direction and it may be plastically deformed (lengthened) to a degree. Therefore, an attempt should be made to shift the IGHL superiorly and medially when repairing the Bankart. This is similar to the T-plasty repair technique of Altchek and associates.[45] Failure to do this may allow the IGHL to sag inferiorly so that the Bankart lesion is not fully repaired.

An arthroscopic grasping instrument is then inserted through the anterior-superior cannula and the IGHL is grasped and shifted superiorly and medially. The drill-guide wire assembly is inserted through the anterior-inferior portal and pushed through the IGHL so that it is close to the glenoid rim between the 4 and 5 o'clock positions (for a right shoulder). It is then drilled to the proper depth and the drill is removed, leaving the guide wire in place (Fig. 43). The bioabsorbable tack is then inserted over the guide wire and impacted so that the IGHL and labrum are securely compressed against the anterior-inferior juxta-articular scapular rim (Fig. 44). Several technical errors can occur with this step. First, the tack may be placed too medially so that the IGHL is not securely fixed at the glenoid edge. Second, the drill can slip either medially along the scapula so that the tack is not securely in bone, or it can slip laterally, injuring the articular cartilage of the joint. Third, the tack can be "button-holed" through the tissue (Fig. 45), or too little tissue can be captured by the head of the tack. Most of these problems can be anticipated and corrected by proper technique. If the tack does "buttonhole," or capture insufficient tissue, it should be left in place and a second tack with better tissue capture should be placed. Removal of the tack from the bone causes bleeding, which may obscure the view for additional surgery. If the tissue of the IGHL is too friable for the tack to gain secure fixation, the procedure should be converted to an open repair.

A second tack is placed above the first one, usually near the 3 o'clock position, and a third tack can be placed at the 2 o'clock position, if necessary. Assessment of the preparation of the glenoid rim and the security of the repair and tack placements is done by viewing through the anterior-superior portal (Fig. 46).

As with all arthroscopic Bankart repair procedures, the shoulder is immobilized in a sling and swathe for 4 weeks. This immobilization time is longer than that of some open capsular repairs that allow range of motion within 10 days and gentle strengthening at 3 weeks. The immediate in vitro strength of this repair has been reported to be 100 N, which is not sufficiently strong to permit immediate range of motion.[44] Patients are permitted to remove their sling to shower after sutures are removed, but they should be instructed to keep the arm either on the abdomen or at the side. At 4 weeks, patients should begin active-assisted range of motion as well as strengthening

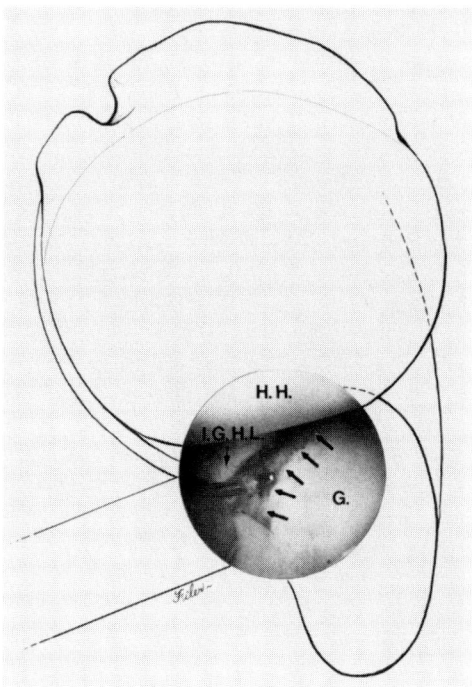 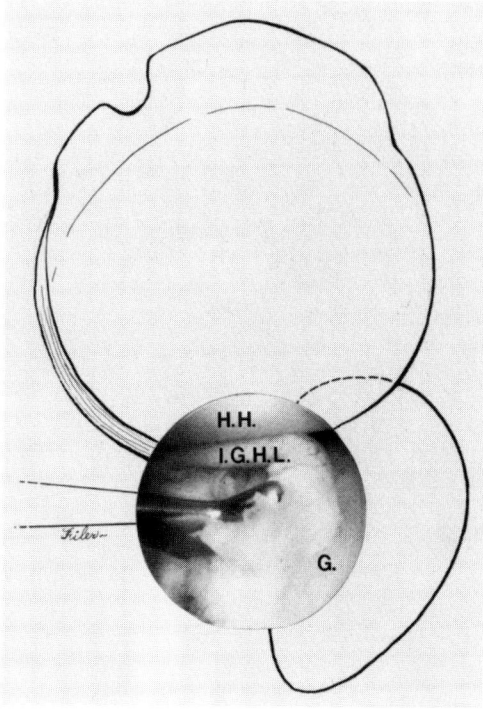

FIGURE 46

Left, Arthroscopic view through the anterior-superior portal of the anterior glenoid rim after preparation prior to Bankart repair. The inferior glenohumeral ligament (IGHL) and humeral head (HH) are labelled for orientation. **Right,** Arthroscopic view through anterior-superior portal after Bankart repair. The Suretac is underneath the arthroscopic probe, and the inferior glenohumeral ligament (IGHL) has been tensioned by the Bankart repair. (Reproduced with permission from Warner JJP, Miller MD, Marks PH, et al: Arthroscopic Bankart repair with the Suretac® device: Part 1. Clinical observations. *Arthroscopy* 1995;11:2-13.)

exercises with elastic bands. Because the limited surgical dissection permits minimal scarring of the soft tissues, motion returns very quickly. At 4 months, strengthening should progress to free weights and isokinetic work (for athletes) and the patient is permitted to toss a ball, swing a tennis racquet for ground strokes (no overhead serving motions), or swim the crawl stroke at half speed. At 6 months, all activities are permitted, except contact and collision sports, which are delayed until 8 to 10 months after surgery.

Clinical Experience With the Suretac® Device

The Suretac device has been used for more than 6 years. Although initial experience (2- to 4-year follow-up)[6] was favorable with a failure rate of 7%, longer follow-up (24 to 60 months) has demonstrated a failure rate approaching that of other techniques (20%).[42] Recent experience with more than 100 cases at another center has shown a failure rate of 7%, although the durability of these results will require longer follow-up analysis.[42] In the seven cases with recurrent shoulder instability, either one of the technical errors previously described had been made, or there was inappropriate patient selection with poor tissue for the arthroscopic repair technique.

Based on this review of these clinical cases, the following recommendations for patient selection and deselection for arthroscopic Bankart repair can be made. First, the history helps the physician determine whether arthroscopic repair techniques are appropriate for the patient. There should be a history of a traumatic injury without any atraumatic or voluntary instability. It can be helpful if there is MRI or CT arthrographic evidence of a Bankart lesion because this suggests that an arthroscopic Bankart repair is a reasonable possibility. Patients with a bony Bankart lesion are often poor candidates because the IGHL is often scarred inferiorly and medially and cannot be mobilized sufficiently for the arthroscopic repair.[36]

The physical examination should not demonstrate hyperlaxity of the shoulder, and the examination under anesthesia should not demonstrate significant inferior (sulcus sign) or posterior translation of the humeral head on the glenoid when a drawer sign is performed in the abducted arm.[45,46] The presence of a Bankart lesion does not necessarily correlate with the degree of perceived shoulder joint laxity.[47] Finally, the patient should be reliable and cooperative and should be willing to comply with the necessary initial postoperative immobilization and limitation of activity.

Second, the patient should have the right tissue. There should be no evidence of an intra-ligamentous injury or ligamentous laxity. The IGHL and other glenohumeral ligaments should be robust and firm when grasped and probed. There should be a discrete Bankart lesion. Associated lesions that have a poor prognosis for this technique include large areas of cartilage loss on the glenoid or humeral head, associated rotator cuff pathology, and large Hill-Sachs lesions. The size of the Hill-Sachs lesion has been associated with recurrent chronic anterior dislocations[48] and the capsuloligamentous structures become stretched and lengthened in these cases. This situation is usually associated with frank anterior dislocation with locking of the humeral head over the glenoid rim on examination under anesthesia. Converting to an open repair permits a capsular shift at the time of the Bankart repair in these patients.

Careful patient selection according to these criteria and meticulous and precise surgical technique will help improve the success of arthroscopic Bankart repair techniques so that they may approach the level currently achieved by open procedures. However, long-term prospective studies based on rigid selection criteria and self-

critical assessment of surgical technique will be necessary to prove the efficacy and effectiveness of these surgical techniques.

An arthroscopic Bankart repair with a bioabsorbable tack can be offered as an option to patients who fulfill the above selection criteria; however, the known higher failure rate compared with open repair techniques must be discussed. The patient must also be informed that there is about a 20% chance that the procedure will be converted to an open technique based on the finding of poor or lax tissue that is not appropriate for arthroscopic fixation. In cases where instability recurs, revision by an open technique is not technically difficult because there is minimal scarring between tissue planes after repair with a tack device.

REFERENCES

1. Griffin LY (ed): *OKU: Sports Medicine.* Rosemont, IL, American Academy of Orthopaedic Surgeons, 1994, pp 93-105.

2. Burkhead WZ Jr, Rockwood CA Jr: Treatment of instability of the shoulder with an exercise program. *J Bone Joint Surg* 1992;74A:890-896.

3. Rowe CR, Patel D, Southmayd WW: The Bankart procedure: A long-term end-result study. *J Bone Joint Surg* 1978;60A:1-16.

4. Arciero RA, Wheeler JH, Ryan JB, et al: Arthroscopic Bankart repair versus nonoperative treatment for acute, initial anterior shoulder dislocations. *Am J Sports Med* 1994;22:589-594.

5. Green MR, Christensen KP: Arthroscopic versus open Bankart procedures: A comparison of early morbidity and complications. *Arthroscopy* 1993;9:371-374.

6. Warner JJP, Warren RF: Arthroscopic Bankart repair using a cannulated, absorbable fixation device. *Op Tech Orthop* 1991;1:192-198.

7. Johnson LL (ed): *Diagnostic and Surgical Arthroscopy of the Shoulder.* St. Louis, MO, Mosby-Year Book, 1993, pp 276-364.

8. Coughlin L, Rubinovich M, Johansson J, et al: Arthroscopic staple capsulorrhaphy for anterior shoulder instability. *Am J Sports Med* 1992;20:253-256.

9. Gross RM: Arthroscopic shoulder capsulorraphy: Does it work? *Am J Sports Med* 1989;17:495-500.

10. Hawkins RB: Arthroscopic stapling repair for shoulder instability: A retrospective study of 50 cases. *Arthroscopy* 1989;5:122-128.

11. Lane JG, Sachs RA, Riehl B: Arthroscopic staple capsulorrhaphy: A long-term follow-up. *Arthroscopy* 1993;9:190-194.

12. Matthews LS, Vetter WL, Oweida SJ, et al: Arthroscopic staple capsulorrhaphy for recurrent anterior shoulder instability. *Arthroscopy* 1988;4:106-111.

13. Committee on Complications of the Arthroscopy Association of North America: Complications in arthroscopy: The knee and other joints. *Arthroscopy* 1986;2:253-258.

14. Wiley AM: Arthroscopy for shoulder instability and a technique for arthroscopic repair. *Arthroscopy* 1988;4:25-30.

15. Wheeler JH, Ryan JB, Arciero RA, et al: Arthroscopic versus nonoperative treatment of acute shoulder dislocations in young athletes. *Arthroscopy* 1989;5:213-217.

16. Burger RS, Shengel D, Bonatus T, et al: Arthroscopic staple capsulorrhaphy for recurrent shoulder instability. *Orthop Trans* 1990;14:596-597.

17. Wilson FD, Adams G, Hile LE, et al: Arthroscopic treatment of the recurrent dislocating shoulder. *Orthop Trans* 1993;17:973.

18. Rao JP, Tovey JE, Zoppi A, et al: Comparison of arthroscopic capsulorrhaphy for anterior shoulder instability: Stapling versus suturing. *Orthop Trans* 1993;17:972-973.

19. Duncan R, Savoie FH III: Arthroscopic inferior capsular shift for multidirectional instability of the shoulder: A preliminary report. *Arthroscopy* 1993;9:24-27.

20. Benedetto KP, Glotzer W: Arthroscopic Bankart procedure by suture technique: Indications, technique, and results. *Arthroscopy* 1992;8:111-115.

21. Caspari RB, Savoie FH: Arthroscopic reconstruction of the shoulder: The Bankart repair, in McGinty JB (ed): *Operative Arthroscopy.* New York, NY, Raven Press, 1991, pp 507-515.

22. Foster CR: Arthroscopic shoulder reconstruction for instability. *Orthop Trans* 1994;18:192.

23. Grana WA, Buckley PD, Yates CK: Arthroscopic Bankart suture repair. *Am J Sports Med* 1993;21:348-353.

24. Goldberg BJ, Nirschl RP, McConnell JP, et al: Arthroscopic transglenoid suture capsulolabral repairs: Preliminary results. *Am J Sports Med* 1993;21:656-665.

25. Geiger DF, Hurley JA, Tovey JA, et al: Results of arthroscopic versus open Bankart suture repair. *Orthop Trans* 1993;17:973.

26. Landsiedl F: Arthroscopic therapy of recurrent anterior luxation of the shoulder by capsular repair. *Arthroscopy* 1992;8:296-304.

27. Neviaser TJ: The anterior labroligamentous periosteal sleeve avulsion lesion: A cause of anterior instability of the shoulder. *Arthroscopy* 1993;9:17-21.

28. Morgan CD, Bodenstab AB: Arthroscopic Bankart suture repair: Technique and early results. *Arthroscopy* 1987;3:111-122.

29. Morgan CD: Arthroscopic transglenoid Bankart suture repair. *Op Tech Orthop* 1991;1:171-179.

30. Maki NJ: Arthroscopic stabilization: Suture technique. *Op Tech Orthop* 1991;1:180-183.

31. Pagnani MJ, Warren RF, Altchek DW, et al: Arthroscopic shoulder stabilization using transglenoid sutures: Four-year minimum follow-up. Proceedings of the 63rd Annual Meeting of the American Academy of Orthopaedic Surgeons, Orlando, FL. Rosemont, IL, 1995, p 131.

32. Rose DJ: Arthroscopic suture capsulorrhaphy for anterior shoulder instability. *Orthop Trans* 1990;14:597.

33. Wolin PM: Arthroscopic glenoid labrum suture repair. *Orthop Trans* 1990;14:597.

34. Wolf EM, Wilk RM, Richmond JC: Arthroscopic Bankart repair using suture anchors. *Op Tech Orthop* 1991;1:184-191.

35. Weber SC: A prospective evaluation comparing arthroscopic and open treatment in the management of recurrent anterior glenohumeral dislocation. *Orthop Trans* 1991;15:763.

36. Walch G, Boileau P, Levigne CH, et al: Arthroscopic stabilization for recurrent anterior shoulder dislocation: Results of 59 cases. *Arthroscopy* 1995;11:173-179.

37. Shea KP, Lovallo JL: Scapulothoracic penetration of a Beath pin: An unusual complication of arthroscopic Bankart suture repair. *Arthroscopy* 1991;7:115-117.

38. Zuckerman JD, Matsen FA III: Complications about the glenohumeral joint related to the use of screws and staples. *J Bone Joint Surg* 1984;66A:175-180.

39. Reider B, Inglis AE: The Bankart procedure modified by the use of prolene pull-out sutures. *J Bone Joint Surg* 1982;64A:628-629.

40. Gerber C, Schneeberger AG, Beck M, et al: Mechanical strength of repairs of the rotator cuff. *J Bone Joint Surg* 1994;76B:371-380.

41. Speer KP, Pagnani M, Warren RF: Arthroscopic anterior shoulder stabilization: 2-5 year follow-up using a bioabsorbable tac. *J Shoulder Elbow Surg* 1995;4(suppl):54.

42. Warner JJP, Miller MD, Marks P, et al: Arthroscopic Bankart repair with the Suretac® device: Part I. Clinical observations. *Arthroscopy* 1995;11:2-13.

43. Speer KP, Warren RF: Arthroscopic shoulder stabilization: A role for biodegradable materials. *Clin Orthop* 1993;291:67-74.

44. Pagnani MJ, Warren RF: Arthroscopic shoulder stabilization. *Op Tech Sports Med* 1993;1:276-284.

45. Altchek DW, Warren RF, Skyhar MJ, et al: T-plasty modification of the Bankart procedure for multidirectional instability of the anterior and inferior types. *J Bone Joint Surg* 1991;73A:105-112.

46. Uhthoff HK, Piscopo M: Anterior capsular redundancy of the shoulder: Congenital or traumatic? An embryological study. *J Bone Joint Surg* 1985;67B:363-366.

47. Speer KP, Deng X, Torzilli PA, et al: A biomechanical evaluation of the Bankart lesion. *Trans Orthop Res Soc* 1993;18:135.

48. Hermodsson I: Röntgenologische Studien über die traumatischen und Habituellen Schultergelenk-verrenhumgen: Nach vorn und Nach Unten. *Acta Radiol* 1934;20(suppl):1-173.

RECURRENT ANTERIOR INSTABILITY: OPEN SURGICAL REPAIR

LOUIS U. BIGLIANI, MD

In the past, numerous open surgical procedures have been described for the repair of anterior glenohumeral instability. The more common of these traditional procedures include repair of the detached glenoid labrum using sutures[1] or staples,[2] muscle transposition of the subscapularis,[3] shortening of the subscapularis and anterior capsule,[4] transfer of the coracoid,[5] osteotomy of the proximal humerus[6] or of the glenoid,[7] and reconstruction using a fascia lata graft.[8] Furthermore, the indication for these procedures was recurrent anterior dislocation and the emphasis for a successful repair was achieving glenohumeral stability. The failure rate for this group of procedures has averaged 3% as measured in terms of recurrence of dislocation. However, as instability repairs are currently evaluated by stricter criteria, which emphasize function and motion as well as stability, there are limitations to a number of these procedures. The loss of motion, especially external rotation, associated with many of these repairs significantly limits overhead activity (such as sports) and has been implicated in the rapid development of postoperative glenohumeral arthritis. Procedures that alter bony anatomy or require metal internal fixation have also become less popular and have been associated with a higher rate of complication.[9,10]

Recently, emphasis has been placed on correcting the specific pathology that is found and restoring normal anatomy rather than distorting anatomy and altering normal shoulder kinematics. An open instability repair should be anatomic, that is, the goal should be to restore the normal capsulolabral anatomic relationships. In most cases, the pathology involves an injury to the IGHL (ie, either detachment from the insertion on the glenoid rim or excessive laxity in the ligament). Bankart[1] described the essential lesion in recurrent instability as detachment of the labrum from the bone and found this pathology in all of his surgical cases. However, recent data have demonstrated that instability can occur without a Bankart lesion or that labral detachment and excessive capsule laxity can coexist (Fig. 47).[11,12] A recent laboratory study on material properties of the IGHL—the principal static restraint against anterior glenohumeral instability—revealed two predominant modes of failure at the glenoid insertion (analogous to a Bankart lesion) and in midsubstance (analogous to capsular stretching and laxity).[13] However, there was significant midsubstance ligament strain before failure, even in the specimens that ultimately failed at the glenoid insertion. These findings are also consistent with the study of arthroscopic findings in acute dislocations, in which all shoulders had grossly visible acute damage to the IGHL, although only 60% had Bankart lesions. Therefore, during a surgical repair, the surgeon should be aware that capsular laxity may also be contributing to the instability lesion. Turkel and associates[14] demonstrated that anterior inferior stability is provided by different regions of the capsule, depending on arm position. As the arm is elevated to a position of abduction and external rotation, the major restraint is the IGHL. Furthermore, Ward and associates[15] recently demonstrated that inferior humeral translation is restrained by the anterior superior capsule and ligaments with the arm at the side and by the inferior capsule and ligaments with the arm in abduction. Therefore, it is important that inferior capsular redundancy also be considered in an anterior repair, because the arm is often used in an abducted externally rotated position. An open anterior instability repair must have the versatility to correct the specific pathology that is encountered at the time of surgery. This pathology may be capsular detachment from the bony rim (Fig. 47, *left*), capsular redundancy anteriorly and inferiorly (Fig. 47, *right*), midsubstance capsular tearing, or capsular detachment from the humeral insertion (a less common lesion).[16]

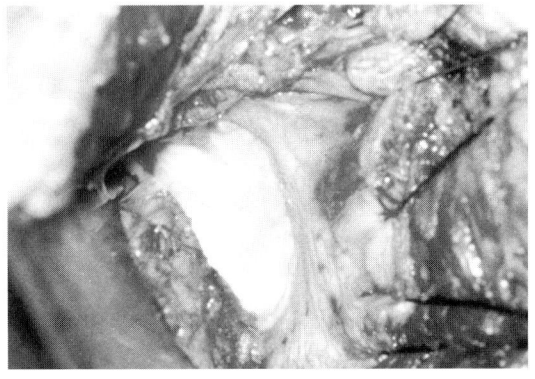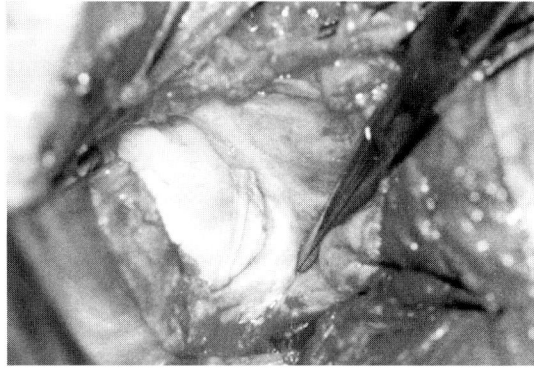

FIGURE 47

A 22-year-old patient with recurrent anterior-inferior instability of the shoulder. **Left,** Patient had an avulsion of the labrum (Bankart lesion) from the anterior and inferior aspect of the glenoid. **Right,** In addition, the patient had a large anterior-inferior pouch secondary to excessive capsular laxity. Therefore, the patient had a combined lesion and surgical repair must combine both aspects of the pathology.

INDICATIONS

The indication for open anterior instability repair is persistent pain and disability secondary to current dislocation or subluxation. Patients usually have had two to three dislocations and are unable to use the arm in an overhead position for work or sports without apprehension. Conservative treatment usually has failed. Open repair offers a reliable method to evaluate and correct the pathology with a high percentage of satisfactory results. Several situations favor open repair over arthroscopic repair, including a large Hill-Sachs lesion, poor quality capsular tissue, return to contact sport, glenoid rim fracture, and inferior capsular laxity. Contraindications to open repair include active infection, a frail extremity secondary to nerve damage, and voluntary instability.

TECHNIQUE

Recently, several different types of repairs have been described that concentrate on correcting primarily capsular pathology. In all of these repairs, the approach to the glenohumeral joint to the level of the subscapularis is a standard that is widely accepted by most authors. The patient is placed in a beach-chair position and an interscalene block is administered. The block is preferred over general anesthesia (Fig. 48) because it pro-

vides excellent muscle relaxation and avoids many of the complications associated with general anesthesia. A concealed anterior axillary skin incision measuring 7 to 8 cm is used (Fig. 49). The subcutaneous layer is mobilized until the inferior aspect of the clavicle is palpated. The cephalic vein is identified and the deltopectoral interval is developed by retracting the cephalic vein laterally with the deltoid muscle. In heavily muscled shoulders, exposure is enhanced by incising the upper portion of the insertion of the pectoralis major, thus allowing easier retraction of the pectoralis muscle. The clavipectoral fascia is incised beginning lateral to the coracoid muscles to avoid damaging the strap muscles, which are gently retracted medially. The coracoid should not be osteotomized because this may lead to injury to the neurovascular structures on the medial side. This maneuver is not routinely needed to enhance exposure. A small wedge of the anterior fascicle of the coracoacromial ligament may be excised in order to allow better visualization of the superior aspect of the subscapularis muscle and the anterior part of the subacromial space. It is important that the upper and lower borders of the subscapularis muscle are identified.

Recently, there has been emphasis on preserving the subscapularis muscle, being careful to repair it in an anatomic position. Most procedures detach the tendinous insertion of the subscapularis muscle in a vertical fashion approximately 1 to 2 cm from the insertion on the lesser tuberosity (Fig. 50).[11,12,17] If the vertical incision is too

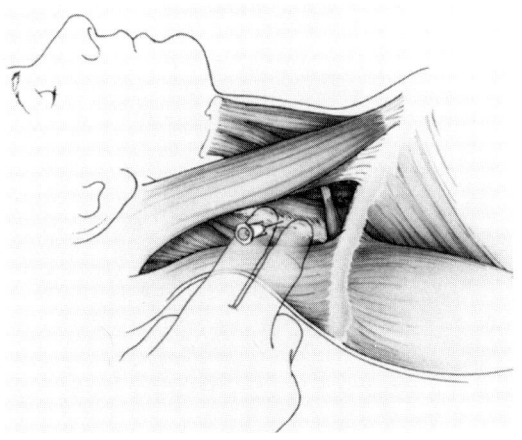

FIGURE 48
Interscalene block anesthesia (regional anesthesia) provides excellent muscle relaxation and anesthesia facilitating the anterior instability repair.

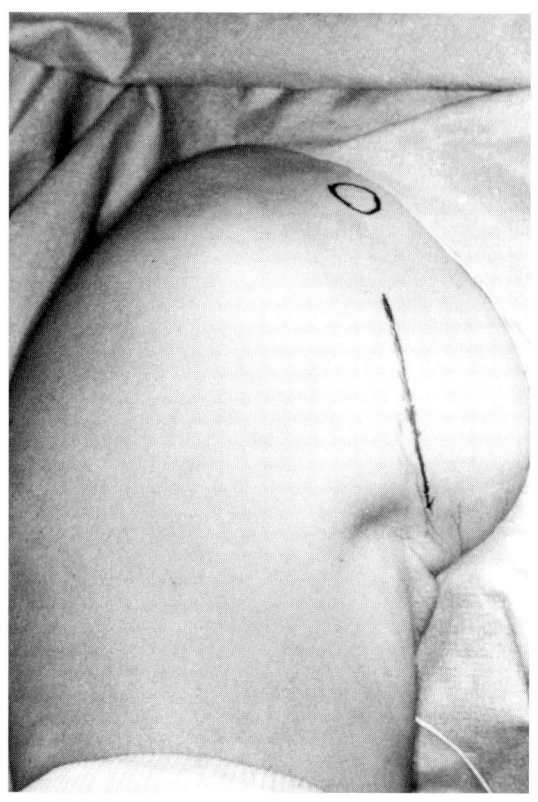

FIGURE 49
A concealed axillary approach provides a very cosmetic scar. The incision starts approximately 3 cm below the tip of the coracoid and extends inferiorly for 8 cm into the axillary recess.

medial, it may damage muscle fibers and compromise the subscapularis repair. It has been suggested that the inferior portion of the subscapularis should be preserved because this will offer protection to the axillary nerve. However, if the inferior portion of the subscapularis is not removed, an inferior capsular dissection may be difficult, if not impossible. An inadequate inferior capsular exposure may compromise the ability to shift the inferior capsule superiorly if there is a significant inferior component to the instability that needs to be corrected. Another approach to the subscapularis muscle has been to split it in a longitudinal fashion in the direction of the muscle fibers.[18] This technique seems to be more appropriate for those procedures that concentrate on correcting the medial capsule and labrum to glenoid rim. Another procedure recommends a vertical, lateral incision in the subscapularis tendon and the capsule as a unit rather than separating the capsule from the subscapularis.[19,20] Only the Bankart lesion is repaired, however, and a capsulorrhaphy is not performed.

Several different types of capsulorrhaphy have been described to address the problem of capsular laxity.[11,12,18,20] These procedures can be classified according to the type of capsular approach to the joint, lateral (humeral), intermediate (middle), or medial (glenoid). These procedures allow

simultaneous repair of a detached anterior inferior labrum and a reduction in joint volume by tightening the capsule and restoring effective functioning of glenohumeral ligaments. The degree of capsular shifting will vary in each case according to the precise amount and location of the excessive capsular laxity encountered. The Bankart lesion must be repaired in addition to shifting the capsule if both lesions are present.

There are several advantages to a lateral capsular incision (Fig. 51). First, more capsule can be shifted. The capsule resembles a funnel with a much broader insertion on the humeral side than on the glenoid side because of the relative differences in circumference. Geometrically, the tissue can be shifted a greater distance and reattached to the broader lateral insertion, thus allowing more tissue to be shifted. This is especially important in shoulders that have inferior laxity in which

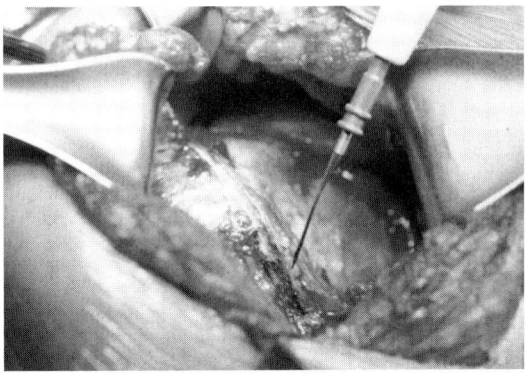
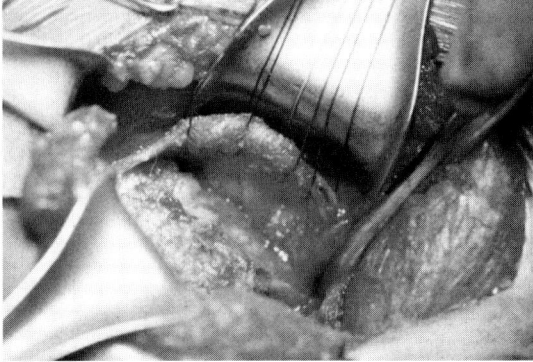

FIGURE 50

The lateral subscapularis approach. **Left,** A cautery is used to make a vertical incision in the subscapularis tendon, approximately 1 cm medial to the lesser tuberosity. **Right,** The subscapularis tendon and muscle is dissected free of the anterior inferior capsule.

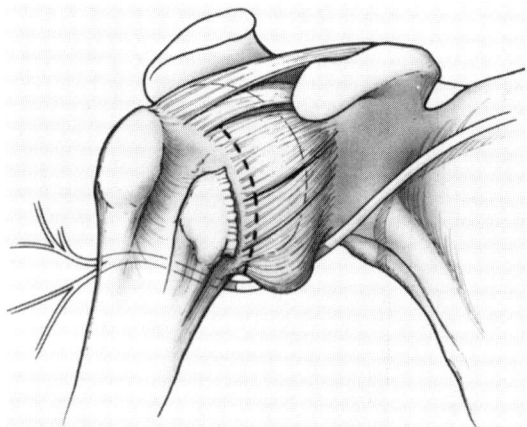

FIGURE 51

A vertical incision is made in the capsule 5 mm medial to the cut made for the subscapularis tendon. The incision begins at the rotator interval.

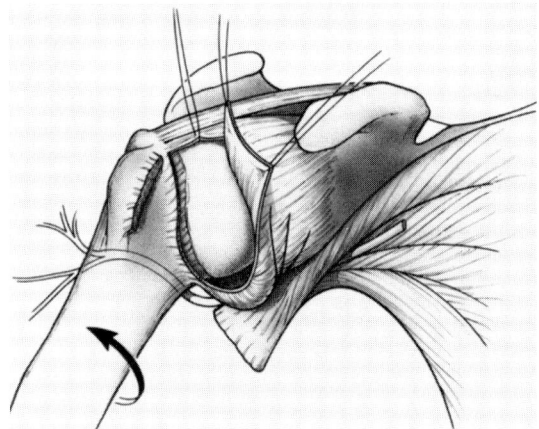

FIGURE 52

The capsule is incised to the neck of the humerus inferiorly on the lateral aspect to protect the axillary nerve. The amount of inferior capsule being detached is dependent on the amount of inferior capsular laxity.

the capsule must be mobilized farther in an inferior direction. With lesser degrees of capsular laxity, the size differential insertion becomes less important. Also, detachment of the capsule laterally affords a degree of protection to the axillary nerve, especially during an inferior dissection when the nerve is at risk as it courses along the undersurface of the midcapsule (Fig. 52). In addition, if the humerus is rotated externally, the capsule insertion is more lateral and the axillary nerve remains in a medial position, providing extra protection. Therefore, it is important to realize that in repairs where the incision is in the midcapsule area, inferior dissection must be done

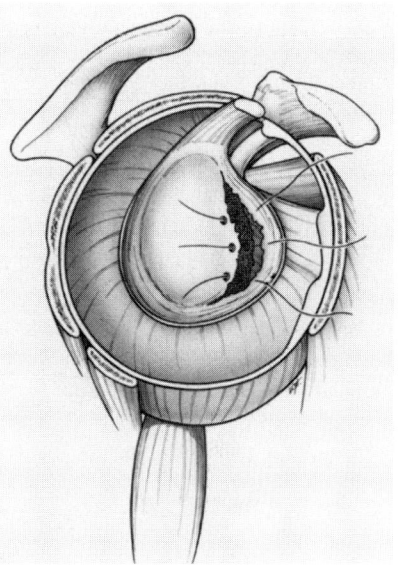

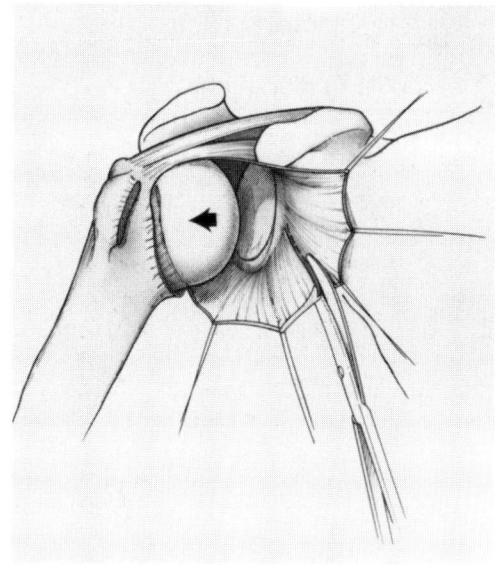

FIGURE 53

A capsulolabral avulsion from the bony neck of the glenoid should be repaired before any attempt at capsulorrhaphy or shifting of the anterior capsule. Bone sutures or suture anchors can be used.

FIGURE 54

A T incision is made in the capsule for a capsular shift. It should be between the inferior glenohumeral ligament and the middle glenohumeral ligament.

very cautiously to avoid injury to the axillary nerve. Finally, capsular tears from the humeral insertion are more readily diagnosed and repaired with a lateral incision. A medial approach to the capsule has the advantage of facilitating a buttress on the glenoid when the capsule is repaired down to the bone. Furthermore, the capsule can be shifted medially and superiorly in this region. This approach also can be done by splitting the subscapularis and not detaching it from its origin on the lesser tuberosity or performing a standard vertical incision at the tendon. During this dissection of the subscapularis and the capsule it is important to evaluate the rotator interval, which may be a source of pathology in recurrent instability. A widened rotator interval can be a significant factor in pathophysiology of recurrent anterior instability. Therefore, it is important to repair the interval as part of an anterior instability reconstruction. However, the interval should not be closed too tight because this may restrict glenohumeral motion, especially external rotation.

When the glenohumeral ligaments and labrum are avulsed medially from the bone, they are reattached to the glenoid rim. The Bankart lesion must be repaired before attempting to shift the

capsule because the capsule must be anchored medially to the glenoid for a shift to be effective. Anchoring the labrum to the bone can be done either by sutures through drill holes in the glenoid rim or by the use of suture anchors (Fig. 53). Two to three drill holes placed close to the articular surface and through the glenoid rim are usually sufficient. Small 4-0 curved curets, curved awes, and heavy towel clips are helpful in making the tunnel. Number 0 nonabsorbable braided nylon sutures are usually sufficient to attach the soft tissue to the bony rim. Sutures may be tied either on the inside or the outside of the capsule; however, sutures tied on the outside decrease the possibility of synovial irritation. Several studies have reported the pull-out strengths of suture anchors and found them to be sufficient to maintain repair of the labrum to the bony rim.[21,22] Depending on the size of the detachment, two to three suture anchors should be placed adjacent to the articular cartilage, but not so medial that a step-off would exist between the glenoid rim and the repaired labrum. The extent of capsular shift depends on the amount of capsular redundancy that is present anteriorly or inferiorly. Because of unidirectional anterior instability, the inferior

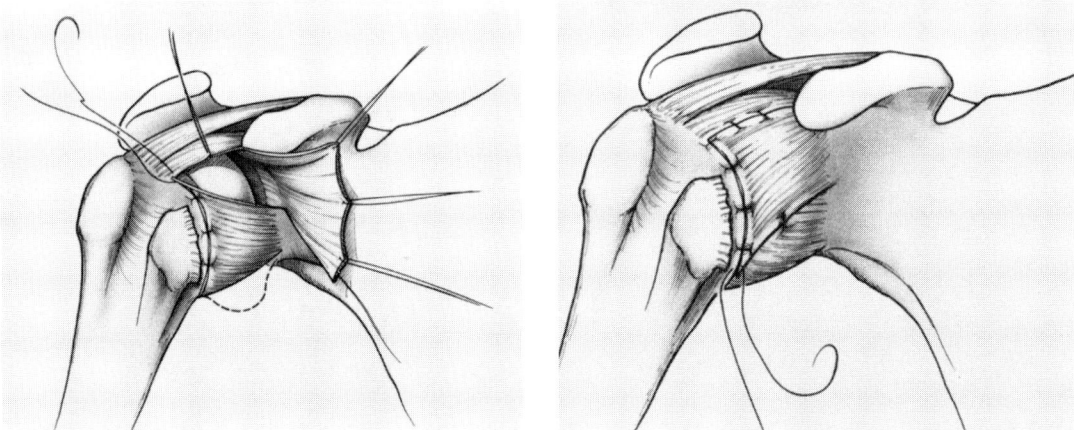

FIGURE 55
Left, The inferior flap is brought up superiorly first to see the tension in the repair with the arm positioned in 20° external rotation and 30° abduction. **Right,** The superior flap is then shifted downward over the inferior flap.

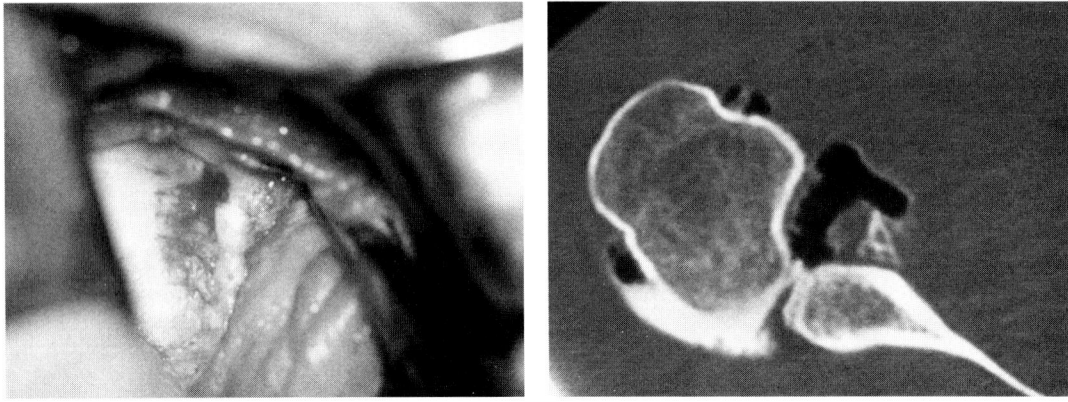

FIGURE 56
Left, Surgical photograph of a patient with a glenoid rim fracture approximately 10% to 15% of the articular surface. **Right,** Computed tomography scan showing the extent of a glenoid rim fracture and the medial displacement.

component is minimal and an inferior shift as well as a T incision in the capsule may not be necessary. However, in cases of inferior capsular redundancy, a T incision should be made in the capsule to allow a superior shift of the inferior capsule. The T incision should be made between the IGHL and MGHL (Fig. 54). The arm should be positioned in at least 20° of external rotation and 30° of abduction during the capsular shift. The inferior part should be shifted superiorly first, fol-

lowed by the superior flap to a more inferior position (Fig. 55). The rotator interval should be loosely closed to avoid overtightening. A stitch may be needed between the superior and inferior flap to enhance conformity.

The pathology in anterior instability also may include anterior glenoid bone deficiency from either a glenoid rim fracture or repeated wear from recurrent dislocation (Fig. 56). Repair of this lesion depends on the location and the size of the

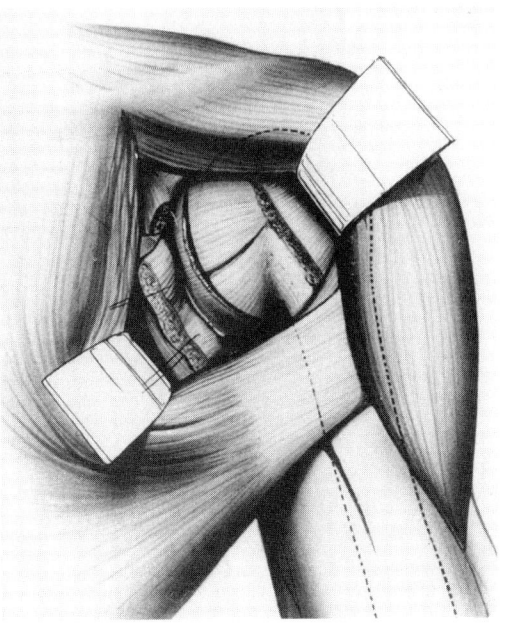

FIGURE 57
An anterior view of the shoulder showing the T-plasty approach, as described by Altchek and Warren. (Reproduced with permission from Altchek DW, Warren RF, Skyhar MJ, et al: T-plasty modification of the Bankart procedure for multidirectional instability of the anterior and inferior types. *J Bone Joint Surg* 1991;73A:105-112.)

glenoid defect. Defects of less than 20% of the surface area of the glenoid can be repaired by suturing the detached labrum back to the edge of the remaining glenoid rim. If a chip of bone has been avulsed with the capsule, the chip of bone should be re-repaired back to the rim of the glenoid. If the fragment is large enough, a cannulated screw can be used, and the screw head can be buried in the substance of the fragment. If the defect is larger than 20% and there is no fracture fragment to be repaired, a bone graft must be used to supplement the anterior rim. The most logical procedure, the Bristow Latarjet procedure, is to transfer the tip of the coracoid with the conjoined tendon of the short head of the biceps and the coracobrachialis muscles.[5] A 4-0 self-tapping malleolar screw is preferable with a washer to avoid fragmenting the coracoid tip. The screw must be long enough to engage the posterior cortex of the glenoid to achieve adequate fixation so that the screw does not pull out. However, it should not protrude too far because this may

cause pain or injury to the suprascapular nerve. The bone graft should be placed very close to the articular edge, within 2 mm, so that a step-off will not be created, leading to recurrent subluxation.[23]

A large Hill-Sachs lesion is another pathologic defect that may require a special technique to gain stability. Treatment options include transfer of the infraspinatus with or without a piece of greater tuberosity into the defect, humeral derotational osteotomy, and increased tightening of the anterior soft-tissue structures to limit external rotation. The simplest option is to tighten the anterior soft-tissue structures, but this maneuver should not excessively restrict external rotation to less than 30° because this will lead to posterior glenoid cartilage wear, posterior subluxation, and osteoarthritic changes.[24]

RESULTS

The recent results that have been reported from the various types of capsulorrhaphies have been encouraging, with a high percentage of satisfactory results in respect to stability, pain relief, range of motion, and function. Satisfactory results have averaged 93%, with an average loss of external rotation of between 5% to 7% and a high percentage return to functional activity, including overhead sports. Rubenstein and associates[18] reported that following an anterior capsular labral reconstruction (medial capsular repair) in 75 athletes, 92% had satisfactory results. Of the professional pitchers in the study, 77% returned to professional competition. Bigliani and associates reported satisfactory results in 59 of 63 athletes having an anterior inferior capsular shift, with 58 (92%) returning to their major sport and 47 (75%) returning to the same competitive level. Altchek and associates[12] reported satisfactory results in 40 of 42 (95%) shoulders undergoing a T-modification of the Bankart procedure (Figs. 57 and 58). However, the medial-based T may require a lateral vertical incision, converting it to an H, to allow further capsular mobilization when there is more inferior laxity. Thomas and Matsen[19] have reported 97% successful results with a surgical approach, incising both the subscapularis and capsule and repairing the Bankart lesion without detaching the subscapularis from the capsule. Berg and Ellison,[20] using a similar type of repair, have reported 89%

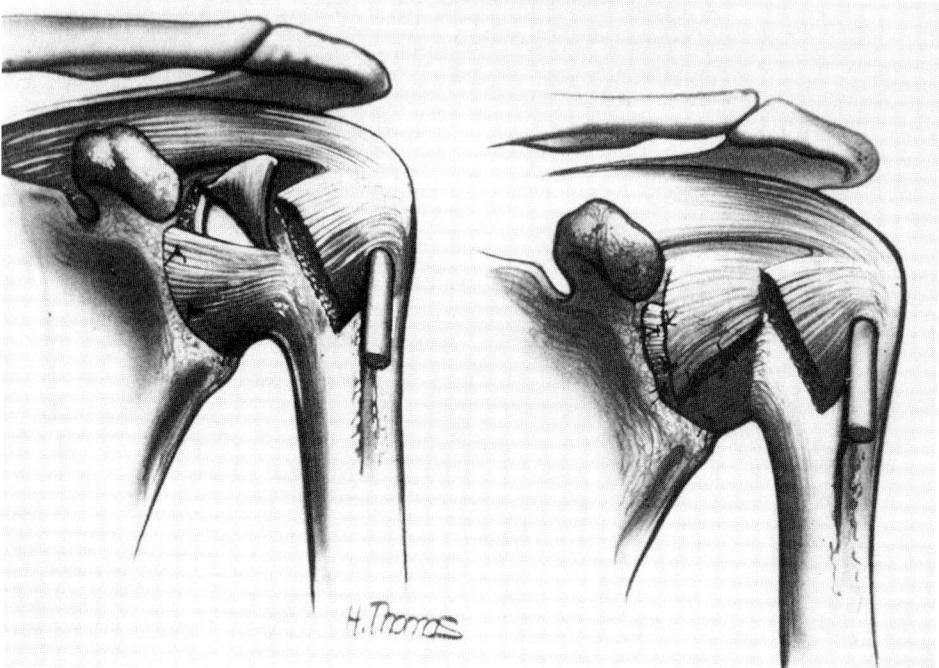

FIGURE 58

T-plasty modification of the Bankart procedure. **Left**, A superior shift of the inferior flap and suture to the glenoid margin. **Right**, The superior flap is to be advanced anteriorly to make a better layered closure. (Reproduced with permission from Altchek DW, Warren RF, Skyhar MJ, et al: T-plasty modification of the Bankart procedure for multidirectional instability of the anterior and inferior types. *J Bone Joint Surg* 1991;73A:105-112.)

satisfactory results. Pollock and associates[25] reported 90% successful results in 151 shoulders undergoing an anterior inferior capsular shift procedure with a redislocation rate of 5%. In another series of 63 athletes having a similar procedure for anterior inferior instability, 94% of patients had satisfactory results. Fifty-eight of 63 (92%) patients returned to their major sport, while 47 (75%) returned to the same competitive level.

Therefore, it appears that procedures which correct the pathology that involves the capsule and labral complex will result in a high percentage of successful results. It is important to remember that the procedure must be versatile enough to correct the specific pathology that is encountered. Multiple lesions may be present in anterior instability involving the labrum, capsule, or anterior bony glenoid rim. A successful open anterior instability repair not only achieves stability but also pain relief and a near-normal range of motion that will allow overhead function.

REFERENCES

1. Bankart ASB: Recurrent or habitual dislocation of the shoulder-joint. *Br Med J* 1923;2:1132-1133.

2. Du Toit GT, Roux D: Recurrent dislocation of the shoulder: A twenty-four year study of the Johannesburg stapling operation. *J Bone Joint Surg* 1956;38A:1-12.

3. Magnuson PB, Stack JK: Recurrent dislocation of the shoulder. *JAMA* 1943;123:889-892.

4. Clarke HO: Habitual dislocation of the shoulder: The Putti-Platt operation. *J Bone Joint Surg* 1948;30B:19-25.

5. Helfet AJ: Coracoid transplantation for recurring dislocation of the shoulder. *J Bone Joint Surg* 1958;40B:198-202.

6. Weber BG, Simpson LA, Hardegger F, et al: Rotational humeral osteotomy for recurrent anterior dislocation of the shoulder associated with a large Hill-Sachs lesion. *J Bone Joint Surg* 1984;66A:1443-1450.

7. Saha AK (ed): *Theory of Shoulder Mechanism: Descriptive and Applied.* Springfield, IL, Charles C Thomas, 1961.

8. Gallie WE, LeMesurier AB: Recurring dislocation of the shoulder. *J Bone Joint Surg* 1948;30B:9-18.

9. Zuckerman JD, Matsen FA III: Complications about the glenohumeral joint related to the use of screws and staples. *J Bone Joint Surg* 1984;66A:175-180.

10. Young DC, Rockwood CA Jr: Complications of a failed Bristow procedure and their management. *J Bone Joint Surg* 1991;73A:969-981.

11. Bigliani LU, Kurzweil PR, Schwartzbach CC, et al: Inferior capsular shift procedure for anterior-inferior shoulder instability in athletes. *Am J Sports Med* 1994;22:578-584.

12. Altchek DW, Warren RF, Skyhar MJ, et al: T-plasty modification of the Bankart procedure for multidirectional instability of the anterior and inferior types. *J Bone Joint Surg* 1991;73A:105-112.

13. Bigliani LU, Pollock RG, Soslowsky LJ, et al: Tensile properties of the inferior glenohumeral ligament. *J Orthop Res* 1992;10:187-197.

14. Turkel SJ, Panio MW, Marshall JL, et al: Stabilizing mechanisms preventing anterior dislocation of the glenohumeral joint. *J Bone Joint Surg* 1981;63A:1208-1217.

15. Ward WG, Bassett FH III, Garrett WE Jr: Anterior staple capsulorrhaphy for recurrent dislocation of the shoulder: A clinical and biomechanical study. *South Med J* 1990;83:510-518.

16. Bach BR, Warren RF, Fronek J: Disruption of the lateral capsule of the shoulder: A cause of recurrent dislocation. *J Bone Joint Surg* 1988;70B:274-276.

17. Bigliani LU: Anterior and posterior capsular shift for multidirectional instability. *Tech Orthop* 1989;3:36-45.

18. Rubenstein DL, Jobe FW, Glousman RE, et al: Anterior capsulolabral reconstruction of the shoulder in athletes. *J Shoulder Elbow Surg* 1992;1:229-237.

19. Thomas SC, Matsen FA III: An approach to the repair of avulsion of the glenohumeral ligaments in the management of traumatic anterior glenohumeral instability. *J Bone Joint Surg* 1989;71A:506-513.

20. Berg EE, Ellison AE: The inside-out Bankart procedure. *Am J Sports Med* 1990;18:129-133.

21. Shea KP, O'Keefe RM Jr, Fulkerson JP: Comparison of initial pull-out strength of arthroscopic suture and staple Bankart repair techniques. *Arthroscopy* 1992;8:179-182.

22. Richmond JC, Donaldson WR, Fu F, et al: Modification of the Bankart reconstruction with a suture anchor: Report of a new technique. *Am J Sports Med* 1991;19:343-346.

23. Hill JA, Lombardo SJ, Kerlan RK, et al: The modified Bristow-Helfet procedure for recurrent anterior shoulder subluxations and dislocations. *Am J Sports Med* 1981;9:283-287.

24. Hawkins RJ, Angelo RL: Glenohumeral osteoarthrosis: A late complication of the Putti-Platt repair. *J Bone Joint Surg* 1990;72A:1193-1197.

25. Pollock RG, Owens JM, Nicholson GP, et al: The anterior inferior capsular shift procedure for anterior glenohumeral instability: Technique and long-term results. *Orthop Trans* 1993-94;17:1109.

POSTERIOR INSTABILITY

ROGER G. POLLOCK, MD

Most authors recommend nonsurgical management of posterior glenohumeral instability as the initial treatment.[1-7] The results of nonsurgical treatment of posterior instability may be superior to the results from nonsurgical treatment of anterior instability. Burkhead and Rockwood,[6] in a study of 140 shoulders with subluxation of various types, found that in each subgroup, patients with posterior instability responded better to exercises than did those with anterior subluxation.[6] Others have been cautious to recommend surgical repair for posterior instability, based on high failure rates with certain surgical procedures. Hawkins and associates,[3] in a retrospective survey of 50 shoulders with posterior instability, urged caution in the selection of patients for surgical repair. In that series, the instability did not appear to be disabling in most of the patients and the results of surgical repair were poor, with a recurrence rate of 50% after surgery.[3] In another recent study, the authors reported a higher degree of satisfaction and ability to return to sports in a conservatively treated group versus a group treated surgically.[7] Optimism about the efficacy of exercises and a somewhat nihilistic view about posterior instability repairs, then, have reinforced the belief in extensive nonsurgical treatment for posterior glenohumeral instability before surgery is contemplated.

However, surgical repair should be considered for those patients with recurrent episodes of posterior instability who continue to have disabling symptoms (pain and loss of function), despite an extensive course of nonsurgical treatment. Patients with voluntary posterior instability must be carefully assessed in order to avoid surgery in those with underlying emotional disorders.[1] This subgroup of patients uses the instability as a means of getting attention and will certainly frustrate efforts at surgical repair. On the other hand, those with the positional type of instability, in which the humeral head subluxes posteriorly when the arm is adducted at 90° of flexion, have responded well to surgical treatment.[1,5,8]

There has been no consensus on when to operate on shoulders with posterior instability, nor has there been a consensus on what procedure to perform when surgery is chosen. Disagreement exists in the literature concerning the underlying pathology of posterior instability. A detachment of the posterior labrum (or reverse Bankart lesion), excessive capsular laxity, a defect of the anterior portion of the humeral head (a reverse Hill-Sachs lesion), increased humeral retroversion and posterior glenoid deficiency (either hypoplasia or excessive retroversion) have all been implicated by various authors.[2,5,7-23] The stabilization procedures can be divided into two groups: those that primarily address bony pathology (either deficient or abnormally directed articular surfaces) and those that correct soft-tissue abnormalities (capsular detachment or excessive laxity).

BONY STABILIZATION PROCEDURES

One procedure for posterior instability repair is based on bony stabilization and employs a posterior bone block, as reported by Hindenach.[12] This procedure is homologous to the Eden-Hybbinette bone block procedure for treating anterior glenohumeral instability.[24-25] Hindenach described the use of this procedure in a patient with atraumatic recurrent posterior instability, in whom the posterior glenoid labrum was found to be intact, but the joint capsule appeared "grossly lax."[12] An iliac graft was fixed to the decorticated surface of the posterior glenoid rim and scapular neck using a Vitallium screw. The graft was positioned so that it projected laterally and extracapsularly for one third of an inch (Fig. 59). The patient had no further episodes of subluxation and follow-up radiographs demonstrated that the iliac graft had been molded to the shape of the humeral head. The author also recommended that a bone block could be used to treat congenital posterior dislo-

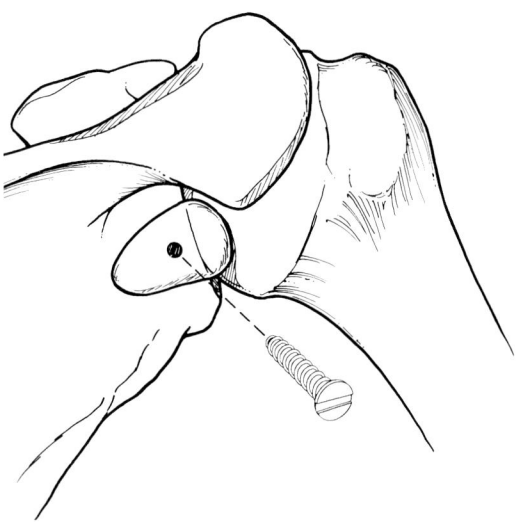

FIG. 59
Stabilization with a posterior bone block. The bone block is fixed to the posterior scapular neck so that it projects past the glenoid margin, extracapsularly. The graft extends the posterior glenoid surface to afford bony stability.

cation, in which the primary lesion is a small glenoid fossa.[12]

Other authors have also described the successful use of a posterior bone block to treat recurrent posterior instability.[5,13,26-28] Fried[27] reported successful treatment with this method in five of six cases. In one case, however, the instability recurred 1 year after surgery and follow-up radiographs demonstrated that the bone graft had been absorbed. Jones[13] reported an excellent outcome in a patient who had been treated with a posterior bone block to salvage a failed soft-tissue repair. In this patient, Jones noted that there was marked laxity of the whole joint capsule and recommended against soft-tissue repairs for this type of posterior instability. Ahlgren and associates[28] reported improvement in stability and a high degree of patient satisfaction in five patients with the iliac bone graft procedure. They emphasized that the graft should be placed in the middle of the posterior aspect of the glenoid, rather than more cranially or caudally.[28] Mowery and associates[26] have recommended combining a posterior bone block with capsular reefing and reported satisfactory results in five patients with this technique. In their technique, the graft

extends 1.5 to 2.0 cm laterally over the humeral head, and it is fixed with a screw that engages the anterior cortex of the glenoid to prevent screw migration. The capsule is then imbricated over the graft so that the bone graft is intracapsular.

The combination of a posterior bone block with a posterior capsular plication had been advocated by McLaughlin[10] for recurrent posterior subluxations of the shoulder. Whereas he had originally recommended a transposition of the subscapularis tendon through an anterior approach for all posterior instability,[9] McLaughlin later reserved this treatment for fixed posterior dislocations, in which there was a defect in the anteromedial portion of the humeral head, into which the tendon could be placed. For recurrent posterior subluxations, a subscapularis transfer had not been effective and posterior capsular plication and bone block were recommended for this condition.[10] More recently, Fronek and associates[5] added a bone block to their capsulorrhaphy procedure when the osseous rim of the posterior glenoid was deficient or when there was severe attenuation of the posterior capsule or infraspinatus. This technique was used in five of their 11 surgically treated cases. These authors harvested the bone graft from the scapular spine, which avoided a second incision and donor site morbidity at the iliac crest. They emphasized that the graft should increase the posterior surface of the glenoid, but that the humeral head should not directly impinge on the graft. The graft is positioned on the posteroinferior quadrant of the glenoid in an extracapsular position to avoid the potential for arthritic changes from the humeral head directly contacting the bone graft. Bigliani and associates[15] and Pollock and Bigliani[29] also combined the use of a capsulorrhaphy with a scapular bone graft, but have reserved the use of bone grafting for unusual cases, in which there is significant glenoid hypoplasia, or for revision cases, in which a previous capsulorrhaphy failed and the remaining soft tissues were deficient.

A second type of repair aimed at providing bony stability in patients with recurrent posterior glenohumeral instability is the opening wedge osteotomy of the scapular neck, or glenoidplasty, and was introduced by Scott.[30] Scott's rationale for this procedure was to provide better stability by reorienting the glenoid, similar to the manner in which acetabuloplasty procedures are used to produce a buttress for congenitally dislocated hips. Several authors have reported that shoulders with posterior instability demonstrate excessive glenoid retroversion, as measured by axial radiographs[18,19,31] or CT scans.[7] These authors have regarded this excessive retroversion as a developmental deformity, predisposing these shoulders to posterior instability. By reorienting the glenoid articular surface to a more normal version, it is suggested that stability can be restored.[18,19,32]

In the original description of the procedure, Scott recommended osteotomizing the posteroinferior aspect of the acromion to provide exposure to the posterior joint. A vertical capsulotomy was performed just lateral to the glenoid rim. If the labrum was detached, the capsule was retracted medially and the osteotomy was performed intracapsularly. If the labrum and capsule were attached to the glenoid rim and scapular neck, the osteotomy was performed through the capsule medial to the glenoid rim. The osteotomy site was then opened, levering the posterior glenoid fragment forward and filling the defect with the osteotomized piece of acromial bone to maintain the reoriented position (Fig. 60). Hardware was not needed to maintain the bone fragment in place in that series. Scott reported satisfactory results with this procedure in two of three shoulders. In the third case, the shoulder dislocated anteriorly in the immediate postoperative period.[30]

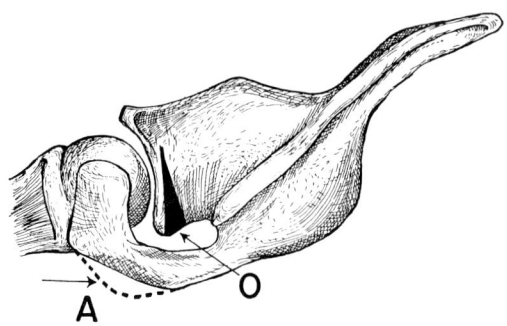

FIG. 60
Glenoid osteotomy (glenoplasty). A portion of the acromion is removed during the exposure and used as a bone graft (A). The black wedge-shaped area represents the osteotomy site that is wedged open (O). The posterior glenoid fragment is levered forward and the defect is filled with the osteotomized piece of acromial bone. (Reproduced with permission from Scott DJ Jr: Treatment of recurrent posterior dislocations of the shoulder by glenoplasty: Report of three cases. *J Bone Joint Surg* 1967;49A:471-476.)

English and Macnab[19] reported success in four patients treated with an opening wedge osteotomy of the glenoid neck, compared with success in only one of four treated with posterior capsulorrhaphy. These authors harvested bone from the spine of the scapula in order to fill the gap made by the opening wedge osteotomy. Brewer and associates[18] reported satisfactory results in four of five shoulders, but revision was necessary to gain stability in one case.[18] These authors chose to use fixation of an iliac graft into the defect of the gap, using one or two centrally placed cortical screws that pass through the wedge graft into the anterior neck of the scapula. They also advocated imbricating the posterior part of the capsule and rotator cuff tendons. Similarly, Hernandez and Drez[16] have recommended combining glenoidplasty with capsular reefing and infraspinatus advancement and have reported generally satisfactory results in eight shoulders treated in this manner.

In two larger series of posterior instability treated with glenoid osteotomy, Wilkinson and Thomas[31] reported recurrence in four of 21 shoulders (14%), while Norwood and Terry[33] found that only ten of 19 shoulders (53%) were stable at follow-up evaluation. Norwood and Terry achieved success in a higher percentage (67%), when the posterior instability was caused by direct trauma. However, the procedure was ineffective in shoulders where the posterior instability is secondary to throwing or swinging (repetitive microtrauma) or to congenital ligamentous laxity.[33] These results suggest that the procedure is more effective for unidirectional posterior instability than for posteroinferior or multidirectional types.

Several other criticisms have been directed at the glenoidplasty procedure. Mowery and associates[26] point out that it is a technically difficult procedure to perform, with respect to creating the osteotomy and shaping the interposed graft. Intraarticular glenoid fracture, nonunion, and loss of graft position may occur with this procedure. Hawkins and associates[3] reported complications in five of 17 shoulders (29%) and recurrence in seven of 17 shoulders (41%) that had been treated for posterior instability with an opening wedge osteotomy of the glenoid. Osteonecrosis of the glenoid due to a shallow osteotomy cut and degenerative arthritis of the glenohumeral joint were among the serious complications in that group of patients. Gerber and associates[34] demonstrated that posterior glenoidplasty pushes the humeral head forward and can cause symptomatic impingement of the anterior rotator cuff between the humeral head and the coracoid process, which these authors have referred to as subcoracoid impingement. Also, the theoretical need to alter the version of the glenoid in most cases of posterior instability has been questioned.[8,26,34] Recent radiographic studies using an axillary view or CT have not demonstrated significant differences in glenoid version between normal and unstable shoulders.[35,36] Other anatomic[26] and radiographic[8,34] studies, which have addressed the specific issue of glenoid version in posterior instability, have also reported only rare cases in which increased retroversion may be implicated as an etiology of this condition.

A third type of bony stabilization procedure for treating recurrent posterior instability is a rotational osteotomy of the humerus. Increased retroversion of the proximal humerus has been cited as a cause of posterior instability and rotation osteotomy has been described to address this problem.[21,37] Chaudhuri and associates[37] reported on 16 humeral osteotomies for recurrent glenohumeral instability, of which 15 cases involved anterior instability. In one case, the osteotomy was performed for recurrent posterior instability. In that case, after the transverse osteotomy had been made in the shaft of the humerus, the distal fragment was rotated externally by 25° and a compression plate was used to facilitate union at the osteotomy site. The authors reported that this shoulder later sustained recurrent anterior dislocations and required further surgery to achieve stability.

Surin and associates[21] reported on 12 shoulders treated with an external rotational osteotomy of the humerus for posterior instability. They used a surgical technique similar to that of Weber and associates,[38] who had reported on rotational osteotomy as a treatment for recurrent anterior instability, but in this series the rotation of the proximal fragment is reversed. Surin and associates recommend performing the osteotomy through cancellous bone just distal to the humeral head, to facilitate healing. The humeral head fragment is rotated 30° externally so that it will no longer slip over the glenoid rim with internal rotation of the arm. Fixation is achieved by the use of an A-O compression plate and screws. The authors reported that stability was achieved in 11 of 12 cases (92%). One patient with multidirectional instability

had recurrent instability and one patient had a nonunion at the osteotomy site, requiring later bone grafting. Most of these shoulders had significant limitation of external rotation after surgery. A second operation for hardware removal was usually performed 1 year after the osteotomy.

SOFT-TISSUE STABILIZATION PROCEDURES

One of the earlier soft-tissue repairs for posterior instability involves repair of a detached posterior labrum and capsule, as described by Rowe and Yee.[39] The authors reported on a posterior approach to the glenohumeral joint in two shoulders, in which the detached capsule was repaired back to the glenoid rim using sutures passed through bone. Their technique resembles that described by Bankart for repair of a detached anterior inferior glenoid labrum. Successful results were achieved in both patients, who were able to return to heavy manual labor. Tibone and associates[14] reported on a series of ten patients treated with a posterior staple capsulorrhaphy, in which a posterior Bankart-type lesion was repaired back to the glenoid rim. Whereas Rowe and Yee had detached the tendinous attachment of the infraspinatus one half inch from its insertion on the greater tuberosity, Tibone and associates developed the interval between the infraspinatus and teres minor without detaching the infraspinatus. A horizontal or transverse arthrotomy was then made through the posterior capsule, which was then pulled medially and fixed with a staple adjacent to the posterior labrum. Three of the ten patients (30%) had postoperative recurrence of the instability, and four had postoperative complications, including a painful staple in one patient, postoperative adhesions in another, and ectopic bone formation in two others. None of these athletes returned to their previous throwing ability, and most complained of a loss of velocity.[14] In a later review of 20 athletes who had undergone posterior staple capsulorrhaphy, Tibone and Ting[40] reported unsatisfactory results in nine patients (45%): six had recurrent posterior instability and three continued to have moderate or severe pain. External rotation decreased significantly, and only one patient regained his previous throwing ability. The authors state that they have abandoned staple capsulorrhaphy and now perform a Bankart-type posterior capsulorrhaphy using sutures. In another recent review, Tibone and Bradley[41] point out that the high-level athlete with posterior instability must be informed that even if the shoulder is successfully stabilized surgically, the functional results may not allow return to sport at the same competitive level.

Boyd and Sisk[11] combined a posterior capsulorrhaphy with a tendon transfer of the long head of the biceps. In this repair, the tendon is routed around the posterior aspect of the neck of the humerus and is stapled to the posterior glenoid rim with the capsule and labrum. The transferred biceps was believed by the authors to function as a dynamic sling, producing an anteriorly directed force on the humeral head. Boyd and Sisk reported successful results for all nine shoulders in which this procedure was employed. However, because the biceps is generally regarded as an important humeral head depressor and stabilizer, its detachment and transfer are not widely recommended.

A reverse Putti-Platt type repair has also been described for treating posterior glenohumeral instability.[3,7,42] This procedure consists of a posterior capsular plication and overlapping of the infraspinatus tendon. Greenhill[42] reported on the use of a posterior Putti-Platt repair in four shoulders with posterior fracture-subluxations of the shoulder. He recommended that by permanently limiting internal rotation to 45°, capsular plication would prevent recurrence of the subluxation. The procedure was technically easier and recovery of shoulder function had been good in these patients. However, in a review of patients treated for recurrent posterior instability by various methods, Hawkins and associates[3] reported disappointing results with the posterior Putti-Platt repair. Of the six shoulders treated with this method, five had recurrent posterior instability at follow-up. Hurley and associates[7] also found the rate of recurrence to be quite high in shoulders that had been stabilized with a reverse Putti-Platt procedure: 17 of 22 shoulders (75%) had recurrent posterior instability after repair. However, many patients with posterior instability have additional components of instability, not merely unidirectional instability.[1,8,29,43] Thus, a shoulder with posteroinferior or multidirectional instability perhaps would be poorly served by a unidirectional tightening of the posterior soft tissues. Failure to

address a significant inferior capsular redundancy may account for the poor results with the reverse Putti-Platt repair, similar to the way in which standard unidirectional anterior repairs fail in bidirectionally or multidirectionally unstable shoulders.[2]

Neer and Foster[2] described the inferior capsular shift for treating inferior and multidirectional instability of the shoulder. They pointed out that this procedure directly addressed inferior capsular laxity, which may accompany instability in other directions. In this procedure, the capsule is detached from the neck of the humerus and shifted superiorly to obliterate the inferior pouch and capsular redundancy on the side of the surgical approach and also to reduce laxity on the opposite side. The procedure is performed using an approach (anterior or posterior) on the side that is most unstable. This repair has been modified to address instabilities that are unidirectional or bidirectional, in addition to those that are multidirectional.[43-46] For instabilities that may involve fewer than three directions, less of an inferior capsular dissection is usually required and the capsular flaps are overlapped with less shifting of the tissue.

The posterior approach for the capsular shift procedure is chosen when the major direction of the instability is posterior. The direction(s) of the instability are established by the preoperative history and physical examination findings and confirmed by the examination under anesthesia at the time of surgery. When the instability is only posterior or posteroinferior, or when it is multidirectional with dislocations in the posterior direction and only lesser degrees of anterior subluxation, then the capsular shift is performed through a posterior approach. This approach allows more direct access to the most redundant portion of the capsule and allows this side of the capsule to be reinforced or doubled in thickness by the cruciate shifting of the capsular flaps. On the other hand, if the instability is mainly anteroinferior with only lesser posterior subluxation, or when the shoulder dislocates in all three directions (ie, is equally unstable anteriorly and posteriorly), then the capsulorrhaphy is performed through an anterior approach.

To perform the posterior-inferior capsular shift procedure,[2,45] an oblique skin incision is used (10 to 12 cm), directed 60° from the scapular spine, starting over the posterolateral aspect of the acromion (Fig. 61, A). The deltoid is split along a posterolateral raphe for a distance of 4 to 5 cm only, to prevent injury to the axillary nerve.

The deltoid is also partially detached from the scapular spine over a distance of 3 to 4 cm, leaving a cuff of tissue on the spine for later repair (Fig. 61, B). The infraspinatus is differentiated from the supraspinatus superiorly and the teres minor inferiorly. The infraspinatus is then carefully separated from the underlying capsule, medially to the glenoid rim and laterally to its insertion at the greater tuberosity. The infraspinatus is then incised in either of two ways: in an oblique fashion, starting medially in a superficial plane and proceeding laterally and deeply, to create two tendon flaps; or, if the tendon is too thin to accomplish this, the infraspinatus can be incised vertically 1 cm medial to the greater tuberosity.

The posterior capsule is incised 1 cm medial to its insertion on the humerus, starting superiorly and proceeding inferiorly along the humeral neck (Fig. 61, C). As the capsule is opened, nonabsorbable sutures are placed at the free edge to assist in mobilizing the tissue. To determine whether sufficient capsule has been mobilized, the surgeon's index finger is placed into the posteroinferior pouch. If pulling up on the sutures pushes the finger out and obliterates this pouch, then enough mobilization has been accomplished for an effective shift. The extent of the inferior dissection and amount of capsule that it is necessary to shift will depend on the amount and location of capsular laxity present. This, of course, will vary from shoulder to shoulder (ie, less in a unidirectional posterior instability than in a multidirectional type). When a complete posterior labral detachment is found (only 10% to 15% of cases), the capsule is first reattached to the posterior glenoid with nonabsorbable braided sutures through bone. After the capsule has been reanchored medially, the capsular flaps can be shifted. The posterior capsule is then split in T fashion at the posterior midglenoid region, creating superior and inferior flaps. The superior flap is shifted inferiorly and reattached to the cuff of capsule left on the lateral aspect of the humeral neck. The inferior flap is then shifted superiorly to obliterate the inferior pouch and to reinforce the posterior capsule (Fig. 61, D and E). The infraspinatus flaps are then repaired, placing the laterally based segment deep, adjacent to the capsule and the medially based segment in a superficial position, further reinforcing the posterior tissues. A posterior bone graft is rarely used because the bony anatomy is usually normal. A bone graft is used in unusual cases when the glenoid bone is deficient, as in glenoid hypoplasia, or in certain revision situations, when the soft tissues appear to be quite deficient.[29] Postoperatively, the shoulder is immobilized for 6 weeks in a plastic brace with the arm at the side in slight abduction and neutral rotation.

The results with this type of posterior capsulorrhaphy have been satisfactory in a high percentage of cases. In their preliminary study, Neer and Foster[2] reported satisfactory results in all 12 patients with at least 1 year follow-up. Neer[43] later reported that he had performed this repair in 23 patients and was unaware of any recurrences of instability. Bigliani and associates[8] analyzed results with this procedure in 35 shoulders with an average follow-up of 5 years. The posterior inferior capsular shift was found to yield overall satisfactory results in 80%. Recurrence of the instability was seen in four shoulders (11%). Five of the six failures occurred in patients who had undergone previous attempts at surgical stabilization. In this group for whom this procedure represented the primary repair, a satisfactory result was achieved in 23 of 24 patients (96%). Similar rates of success were achieved, regardless of the direction (unidirectional versus bidirectional versus multidirectional) or etiology (traumatic versus atraumatic).[8] Fronek and associates,[5] as previously discussed, also found a high rate of success with posterior capsulorrhaphy in a group of 11 patients. In that series, ten of 11 patients (91%) achieved a satisfactory result, with a medially based capsulorrhaphy alone or with capsulorrhaphy supplemented with a bone graft (Fig. 62). More recently, Santini and Nevaiser[47] reported no further episodes of instability in 16 of 18 shoulders treated with a posterior inferior capsular shift. Only two developed recurrent instability and were rated as failures, while those with satisfactory results regained normal strength and function.

Advocates of the posterior inferior capsular shift point out that it directly addresses the basic pathology that is usually encountered in shoulders with posterior instability, namely, redundancy of the posterior inferior joint capsule. When additional pathology is encountered, such as posterior labral detachment or glenoid deficiency, the procedure can be modified to address these lesions, by incorporating labral re-attachment or posterior bone grafting, respectively, into the capsulorrhaphy.

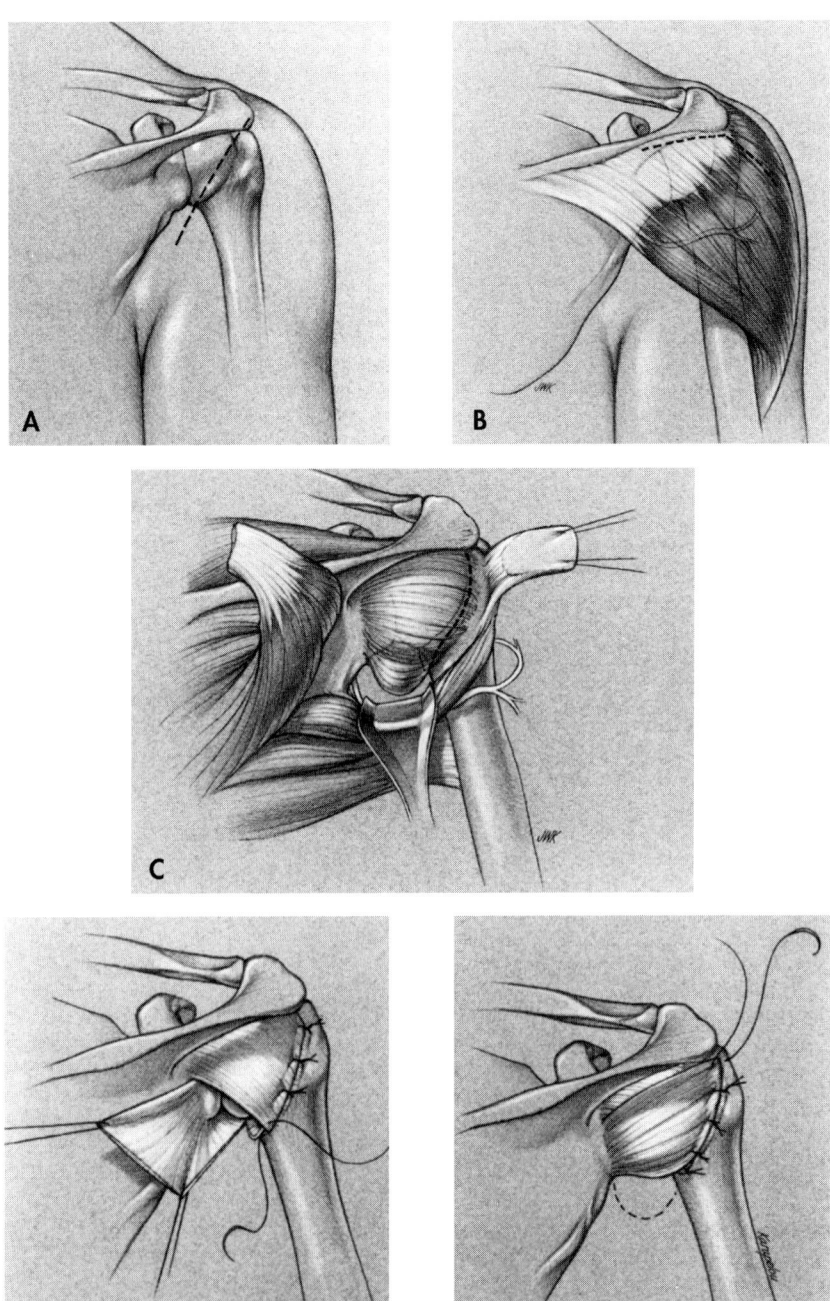

FIG. 61

A, An oblique skin incision is used, directed 60° from the scapular spine. This incision allows for better cosmesis than a transverse incision over the scapular spine. **B,** The deltoid is split in a posterolateral raphe, starting at the posterior acromial tip and proceeding distally for a distance less than 5.0 cm. It is also detached from the scapular spine (3 to 4 cm) to afford exposure. **C,** A capsular incision is made 1 cm medial to its insertion on the humerus, starting superiorly and proceeding inferiorly along the humeral neck. **D,** The superior capsular flap is shifted inferiorly and reattached to the lateral capsular remnant. **E,** The inferior flap is then shifted superiorly and reattached laterally, reducing the inferior capsular redundancy and reinforcing the repair.

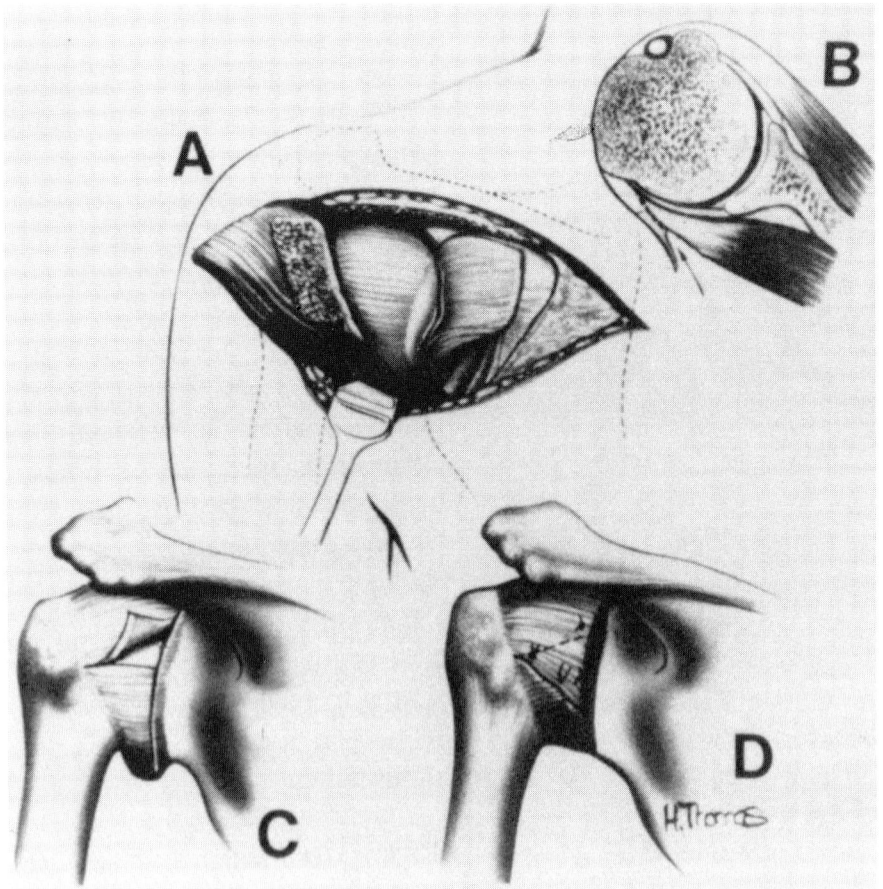

FIG. 62
Medially based posterior capsulorrhaphy. **A,** Deltoid dissection off the scapular spine to expose the underlying posterior rotator cuff tendons. **B,** The infraspinatus tendon is stripped off the capsule at an oblique angle to obtain maximum length. **C,** T-shaped capsular incision at the margin of the glenoid. **D,** Medially based capsulorrhaphy with nonabsorbable sutures. (Reproduced with permission from Fronek J, Warren RF, Bowen M: Posterior subluxation of the glenohumeral joint. *J Bone Joint Surg* 1989;71A:205-216.)

REFERENCES

1. Rowe CR, Pierce DS, Clark JG: Voluntary dislocation of the shoulder: A preliminary report on a clinical, electromyographic, and psychiatric study of twenty-six patients. *J Bone Joint Surg* 1973;55A:445-460.

2. Neer CS II, Foster CR: Inferior capsular shift for involuntary inferior and multidirectional instability of the shoulder: A preliminary report. *J Bone Joint Surg* 1980;62A:897-908.

3. Hawkins RJ, Koppert G, Johnston G: Recurrent posterior instability (subluxation) of the shoulder. *J Bone Joint Surg* 1984;66A:169-174.

4. Jobe FW: The shoulder in sports, in Rockwood CA Jr, Matsen FA III (eds): *The Shoulder.* Philadelphia, PA, WB Saunders, 1990, pp 961-990.

5. Fronek J, Warren RF, Bowen M: Posterior subluxation of the glenohumeral joint. *J Bone Joint Surg* 1989;71A:205-216.

6. Burkhead WZ Jr, Rockwood CA Jr: Treatment of instability of the shoulder with an exercise program. *J Bone Joint Surg* 1992;74A:890-896.

7. Hurley JA, Anderson TE, Dear W, et al: Posterior shoulder instability: Surgical versus conservative results with evaluation of glenoid version. *Am J Sports Med* 1992;20:396-400.

8. Bigliani LU, Pollock RG, McIlveen SJ, et al: Shift of the posteroinferior aspect of the capsule for recurrent posterior glenohumeral instability. *J Bone Joint Surg* 1995;77:1011-1020.

9. McLaughlin HL: Posterior dislocation of the shoulder. *J Bone Joint Surg* 1952;34A:584-590.

10. McLaughlin HL: Follow-up notes on articles previously published in the journal: Posterior dislocation of the shoulder. *J Bone Joint Surg* 1962;44A:1477.

11. Boyd HB, Sisk TD: Recurrent posterior dislocation of the shoulder. *J Bone Joint Surg* 1972;54A:779-786.

12. Hindenach JCR: Recurrent posterior dislocation of the shoulder. *J Bone Joint Surg* 1947;29:582-586.

13. Jones V: Recurrent posterior dislocation of the shoulder: Report of a case treated by posterior bone block. *J Bone Joint Surg* 1958;40B:203-207.

14. Tibone JE, Prietto C, Jobe FW, et al: Staple capsulorrhaphy for recurrent posterior shoulder dislocation. *Am J Sports Med* 1981;9:135-139.

15. Bigliani LU, Endrizzi DP, McIlveen SJ, et al: Operative management of posterior shoulder instability. *Orthop Trans* 1989;13:232.

16. Hernandez A, Drez D: Operative treatment of posterior shoulder dislocations by posterior glenoidplasty, capsulorrhaphy, and infraspinatus advancement. *Am J Sports Med* 1986;14:187-191.

17. Goss TP, Costello G: Works in progress #3: Recurrent symptomatic posterior glenohumeral subluxation. *Orthop Rev* 1988;17:1024-1028,1032.

18. Brewer BJ, Wubben RC, Carrera GF: Excessive retroversion of the glenoid cavity: A cause of non-traumatic posterior instability of the shoulder. *J Bone Joint Surg* 1986;68A:724-731.

19. English E, Macnab I: Recurrent posterior dislocation of the shoulder. *Can J Surg* 1974;17:147-151.

20. Saha AK: Dynamic stability of the glenohumeral joint. *Acta Orthop Scand* 1971;42:491-505.

21. Surin V, Blader S, Markhede G, et al: Rotational osteotomy of the humerus for posterior instability of the shoulder. *J Bone Joint Surg* 1990;72A:181-186.

22. Nobel W: Posterior traumatic dislocation of the shoulder. *J Bone Joint Surg* 1962;44A:523-537.

23. Wilson JC, McKeever FM: Traumatic posterior (retroglenoid) dislocation of the humerus. *J Bone Joint Surg* 1949;31A:160-172.

24. Eden R: Zur operation der habituellen schulterluxation unter mitteilung eines neuen verfahrens bei abriss am inneren pfannenrande. *Dtsch Ztshr Chir* 1918;144:269.

25. Hybbinette S: De la transplantation d'un fragment osseux pout remedier aux luxations recidiântes de l'épaule: Constatations et résultats opératoires. *Acta Chir Scan* 1932;71:411-443.

26. Mowery CA, Garfin SR, Booth RE, et al: Recurrent posterior dislocation of the shoulder: Treatment using a bone block. *J Bone Joint Surg* 1985;67A:777-781.

27. Fried A: Habitual posterior dislocation of the shoulder joint: A report of 15 operated cases. *Acta Orthop Scand* 1949;18:329-345.

28. Ahlgren SA, Hedlund T, Nistor L: Idiopathic posterior instability of the shoulder joint: Results of operation with posterior bone graft. *Acta Orthop Scand* 1978;49:600-603.

29. Pollock RG, Bigliani LU: Recurrent posterior shoulder instability: Diagnosis and treatment. *Clin Orthop* 1993;291:85-96.

30. Scott DJ Jr: Treatment of recurrent posterior dislocations of the shoulder by glenoplasty: Report of three cases. *J Bone Joint Surg* 1967;49A:471-476.

31. Wilkinson JA, Thomas WG: Glenoid osteotomy for recurrent posterior dislocation of the shoulder. *J Bone Joint Surg* 1985;67B:496.

32. Pouget G: Recurrent posterior dislocation of the shoulder treated by glenoid osteotomy. *J Bone Joint Surg* 1984;66B:140.

33. Norwood LA, Terry GC: Shoulder posterior subluxation. *Am J Sports Med* 1984;12:25-30.

34. Gerber C, Ganz R, Vinh TS: Glenoplasty for recurrent posterior shoulder instability: An anatomic reappraisal. *Clin Orthop* 1987;216:70-79.

35. Cyprien JM, Vasey HM, Burdet A, et al: Humeral retrotorsion and glenohumeral relationship in the normal shoulder and in recurrent anterior dislocation (scapulometry). *Clin Orthop* 1983;175:8-17.

36. Randelli M, Gambrioli PL: Glenohumeral osteometry by computed tomography in normal and unstable shoulders. *Clin Orthop* 1986;208:151-156.

37. Chaudhuri GK, Sengupta A, Saha AK: Rotation osteotomy of the shaft of the humerus for recurrent dislocation of the shoulder: Anterior and posterior. *Acta Orthop Scand* 1974;45:193-198.

38. Weber BG, Simpson LA, Hardegger F, et al: Rotational humeral osteotomy for recurrent anterior dislocation of the shoulder associated with a large Hill-Sachs lesion. *J Bone Joint Surg* 1984;66A:1443-1450.

39. Rowe CR, Yee LBK: A posterior approach to the shoulder joint. *J Bone Joint Surg* 1944;26A:580-584.

40. Tibone J, Ting A: Capsulorrhaphy with a staple for recurrent posterior subluxation of the shoulder. *J Bone Joint Surg* 1990;72A:999-1002.

41. Tibone JE, Bradley JP: The treatment of posterior subluxation in athletes. *Clin Orthop* 1993;291:124-137.

42. Greenhill BJ: Persistent posterior shoulder dislocation: Its diagnosis and its treatment by posterior Putti-Platt repair. *J Bone Joint Surg* 1972;54B:763.

43. Neer CS II (ed): *Shoulder Reconstruction.* Philadelphia, PA, WB Saunders, 1990.

44. Neer CS II, Fithian TE, Hansen PE, et al: Reinforced cruciate repair for anterior dislocation of the shoulder. *Orthop Trans* 1985;9:44.

45. Bigliani LU: Anterior and posterior capsular shift for multidirectional instability. *Tech Orthop* 1989;3:36-45.

46. Pollock RG, Owens JM, Nicholson GP, et al: The anterior inferior capsular shift procedure for glenohumeral instability. *Orthop Trans* 1994;18:974.

47. Santini A, Nevaiser R: Long term results of posterior inferior capsular shift. *J Shoulder Elbow Surg* 1995;4(suppl):S65

MULTIDIRECTIONAL INSTABILITY

EVAN L. FLATOW, MD

Much of the historic literature on glenohumeral instability concerned recurrent, locked, anterior glenohumeral dislocations. The situation became understandably more complex with the addition of subluxation as a category of instability, and with the appreciation that symptomatic glenohumeral translations could occur in multiple directions. In 1980, Neer and Foster[1] noted that few articles had as yet been written about the treatment of inferior and multidirectional instability of the shoulder. Citing the work of Endo, Bateman,[2] DePalma,[3] Rowe and associates,[4] and Thompson and associates (unpublished data, 1965), they noted that while authors agreed on the need to distinguish this disorder from routine unidirectional dislocations (and from voluntary dislocations) and on the importance of allowing a thorough trial of strengthening exercises before considering surgical treatment, there was little consensus as to the best method of reconstruction.

In introducing inferior capsular shift as a treatment for involuntary inferior and multidirectional instability, Neer[1,5] emphasized five key points. (1) Loose shoulders are often without pain, and the surgeon must be convinced that the instability is symptomatic before considering repair. (2) In addition to major trauma and inherent ligamentous laxity, acquired shoulder laxity from repetitive minor injury and stress (as in swimming the butterfly stroke or in gymnastics) is often an important factor in the development of multidirectional instability. (3) Unidirectional surgical procedures may fail in multidirectional patients because they incompletely correct the instability (eg, not addressing inferior and posterior components that remain symptomatic) and because they can asymmetrically tighten the joint, causing a fixed subluxation to the opposite side, which can result in arthritis. (4) Hyperlaxity of the capsule with excessive joint volume must be corrected by globally tensioning the capsule anteriorly, inferiorly, and posteriorly, while thickening and reinforcing it on the side of greatest instability (anterior or posterior).

(5) Rehabilitation of the muscles that stabilize the humerus is important not only in nonsurgical management, but in protecting the repair postoperatively, "as the capsule and ligaments normally function only as a checkrein."[1]

In the ensuing 15 years it has become evident that misdiagnosis or improper treatment of multidirectional instability is a significant cause of clinical failure.[6-18] It is especially tragic when asymmetric tightening of one side of a hypermobile joint causes glenohumeral arthritis, often at a very young age.[10,13,17-20] Conversely, appropriate evaluation and treatment leads to satisfactory results in a high proportion of patients with multidirectional instability.[1,7,8,21-27]

DEFINITION

Patients with multidirectional instability have symptomatic glenohumeral instability in more than one direction: anterior, inferior, and posterior.[1,24,28] Several areas of confusion have, however, developed around this seemingly straightforward definition.[29,30]

(1) Routine unidirectional anterior instability actually involves *anteroinferior* dislocations because the coracoid blocks straight anterior dislocation. However, this is not the same as having instability both anteriorly and inferiorly; such a patient will have an additional element of straight inferior instability evident as a "sulcus" sign, with the arm at the side and an inferior sag of the humerus with the arm abducted.

(2) Some authors have taken Neer's warning that not all loose shoulders are symptomatic (eg, a loose shoulder may have pain not due to instability but to unrecognized acromioclavicular pain) a step farther by suggesting that there may be elements of asymptomatic laxity and

symptomatic instability in the same shoulder (eg, a shoulder with "normal" inferior and posterior laxity but symptomatic anterior instability).[29-31] However, the clinical value of making this distinction (and a reliable method of effecting it) has never been established, while the problems associated with performing a unidirectional operation on a multidirectional shoulder have been well documented.

(3) There has been controversy as to whether multidirectional instability is a completely separate condition from unidirectional, recurrent instability, or just the other end of a "laxity spectrum." Bigliani and associates[32] found that anterior instability in athletes constituted a spectrum from unidirectional anterior instability to frank multidirectional instability, with pronounced inferior capsular laxity. For this reason, they used an inferior capsular shift approach[1] in all cases, modifying the repair as needed to correct the specific degree of capsular laxity found in each instance.

ETIOLOGY

There is a common misconception that multidirectional instability is limited to young sedentary patients with generalized ligamentous laxity who often present with bilateral symptoms and signs (Fig. 63). Furthermore, the instability is classically thought of as being acquired in an atraumatic fashion. Although there is a group of such patients, shoulders with multidirectional instability are often found in athletic patients, many of whom have had significant injuries.[13] Repetitive microtrauma, seen for example in butterfly swimming or in gymnastics, can also lead to multidirectional instability by selectively "stretching out" shoulders in comparison to other joints, which may not be lax on examination (Fig. 64). Additionally, shoulders with multidirectional instability may have Bankart lesions[21] and humeral head impression defects,[13] although less commonly than unidirectional cases resulting from hard trauma.

Although statistical generalizations may be helpful in education and in raising the level of suspicion of multidirectional instability in patients in whom an associated finding is dis-

covered, they can be dangerous if they are interpreted as strict guidelines for diagnosis. It is precisely the "overlap" patient who is most likely to be misdiagnosed.

CLINICAL PRESENTATION

Patients with multidirectional instability may present in a variety of ways. While extremely hypermobile shoulders can become symptomatic without unusual trauma and possibly even from the activities of daily living, the patient is often athletic; swimmers, weightlifters, and gymnasts may be particularly predisposed to instability. A common presentation appears to be an individual with a relatively loose shoulder who stresses it repetitively in athletic activities or work-related events. A dislocation may have occurred without significant injury and spontaneously reduced or self reduced.

Symptoms may suggest the directions of instability involved. Inferior instability may present with pain associated with carrying heavy suitcases or shopping bags. Occasionally, these symptoms are accompanied by traction (brachial plexus) paresthesias. Pain associated with pushing open heavy doors or use of the arm in a forward flexed and internally rotated position usually suggests a component of posterior instability, while discomfort in the overhead, abducted and externally rotated position tends to implicate anterior instability. However, symptoms can be complex, vague, and difficult to sort out.

There may be a family history of loose joints or ligamentous laxity. Biochemical abnormalities, generalized laxity syndromes, and relationships to defined collagen disorders (eg, Ehlers-Danlos) have been investigated but not well characterized.[33-40] It is important to carefully evaluate each patient's history for suggestions of voluntary instability.

The physical examination may demonstrate evidence of generalized ligamentous laxity, such as hyperextension at the elbows, the ability to approximate the thumbs to the forearms, hyperextension of the metacarpophalangeal joints, or patellofemoral subluxation. In some of these patients we have noted hypermobile acromioclavicular and sternoclavicular joints, which can be sources of symptoms. It is important, there-

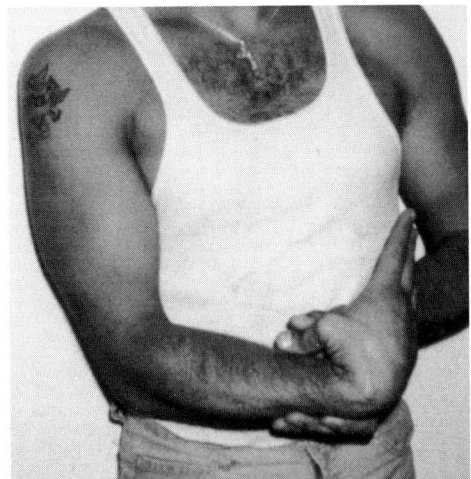
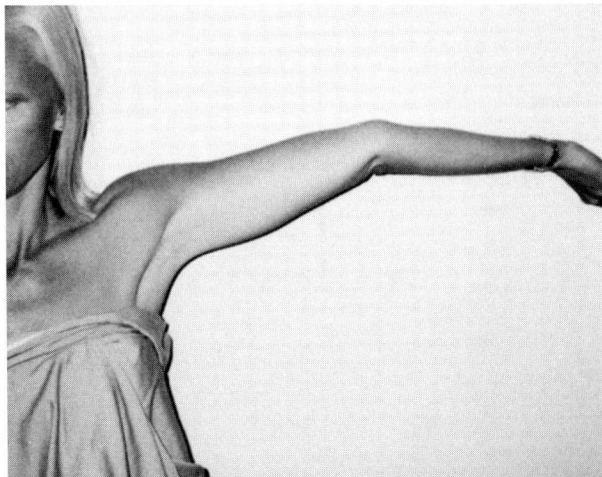
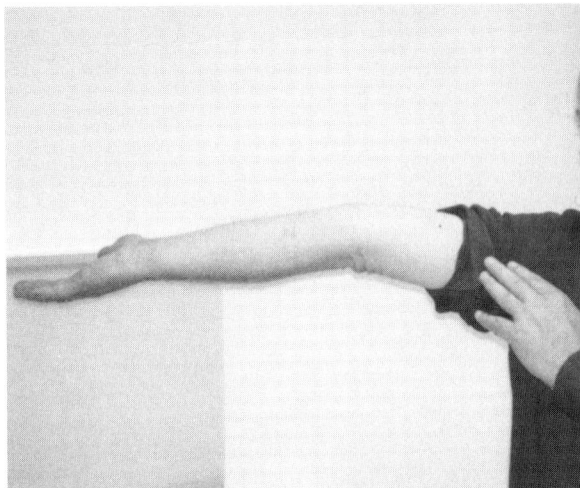
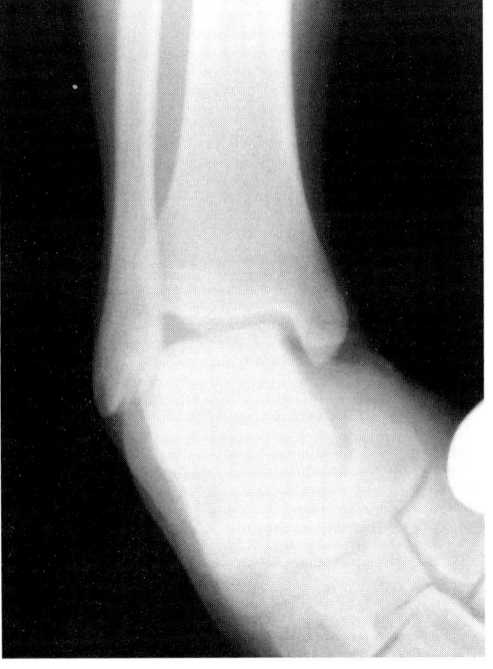

FIGURE 63
Generalized ligamentous laxity. **Top left,** Laxity of the thumb is demonstrated in this patient. He can approximate his thumb to his forearm. **Top right,** Laxity of the elbow is demonstrated in this patient. She can hyperextend her elbow. **Bottom left,** Generalized laxity often runs in families. Laxity of the elbow is demonstrated in the father of a patient with multidirectional instability. The patient's younger brother can "pop" his shoulders "in and out," the patient's paternal grandmother can "flip her joints around," and the patient's paternal aunt can "do strange things with her knees." **Bottom right,** Stress radiograph of the ankle of a patient with multidirectional instability. In addition to shoulder surgery, he required bilateral ankle reconstructions for chronic instability after numerous athletic injuries.

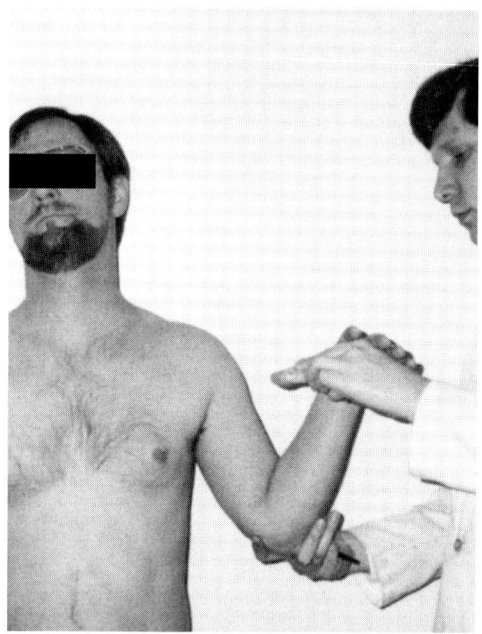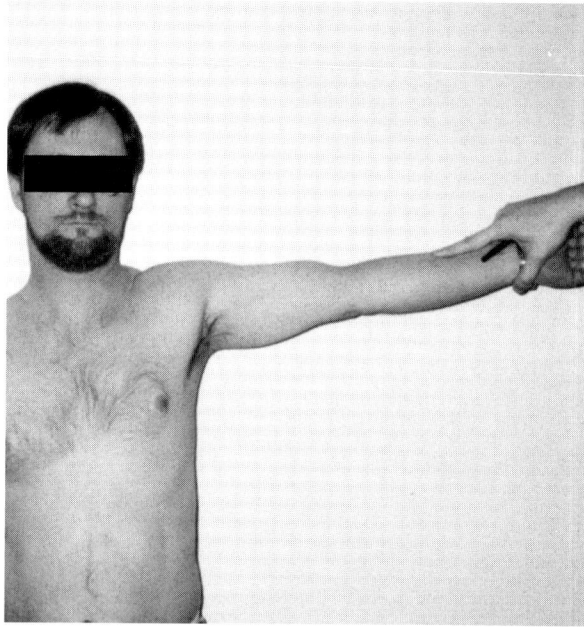

FIGURE 64

Acquired shoulder laxity. **Left,** This patient had multidirectional shoulder instability. He has a history of extensive gymnastics during youth, including the rings. Although his shoulders were stretched out over years of repetitive microtrauma, he does not have thumb laxity. **Right,** Patient does not have elbow laxity.

fore, to examine these joints for tenderness. The most significant finding, however, is the ability to sublux the glenohumeral joint in multiple directions with the reproduction of the patient's usual pain. The sulcus sign (inferior sag of the humerus with the arm at the side) and inferior translation of the abducted humerus are especially helpful in elucidating inferior laxity (Fig. 65).

Additionally, close inspection of the scapulothoracic articulation should be performed because concomitant scapulothoracic instability may occasionally be present.[13,41] There may be multiple positive findings using the following maneuvers: anterior and posterior load and shift tests, anterior and posterior apprehension tests, the fulcrum test, relocation test, Fukuda test, and the push-pull or supine stress test.[1,13,41,42] The aim is to produce humeral translations either anteriorly, posteriorly, or inferiorly (relative to the glenoid), and to document that these translations are reliably accompanied by the patient's report of the usual pain and discomfort. Laxity may be asymptomatic but dramatic enough to distract the examiner from the primary source of pain, such

as a painful acromioclavicular joint or a cervical radiculopathy. Conversely, laxity may be hard to demonstrate, even in a shoulder with multidirectional instability, if pain, muscle spasm, and guarding prevent subluxation. It is helpful to examine the contralateral, asymptomatic shoulder for laxity. If it is extremely loose it may be a clue to the multidirectional nature of the affected side.

It can be difficult to determine the primary direction of instability on physical examination. Determining whether the shoulder is moving from a dislocated to a reduced position or from a reduced to a dislocated position can be challenging. Maintaining the fingers of one hand on the coracoid anteriorly and the posterolateral acromion can aid in this determination. For this reason, multiple physical examinations on different days are frequently helpful in assessing these patients.[25]

Plain radiographs are generally normal but should be evaluated for the presence of humeral head defects and/or glenoid lesions, such as osseous Bankart fragments, reactive bone, or wear. Regular or CT arthrograms may demon-

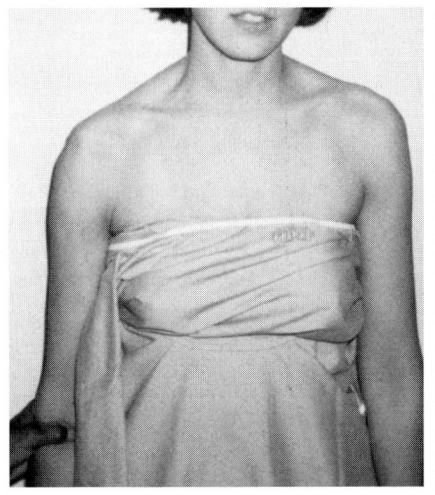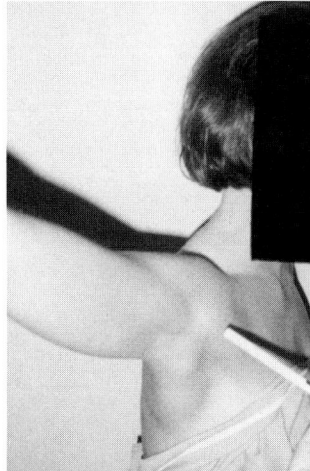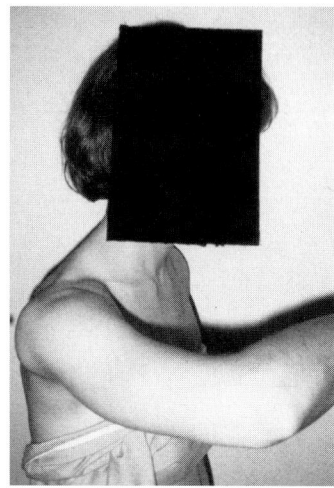

FIGURE 65
Multidirectional instability treated by inferior capsular shift from a posterior approach. **Left,** This is a 22-year-old female with a 3+ sulcus sign as her arm is pulled. **Center,** She subluxes anteriorly with her arm extended and externally rotated. This is symptomatic and prevents overhead activities. **Right,** She dislocates posteriorly with her arm flexed and internally rotated, and she is unable to reach for objects or push open doors.

strate an increased capsular volume (Fig. 66) and, less commonly, labral detachments. MRI is less satisfactory in demonstrating the redundant capsule because of the lack of joint distention; however, labral lesions can be detected if present. Stress radiographs can demonstrate laxity, especially inferior subluxation, but are not generally needed.[43] Cine MRI is currently investigational but has the potential to dynamically demonstrate capsular and labral defects in varying positions.[44]

NONSURGICAL MANAGEMENT

Once the diagnosis of multidirectional instability has been established, a prolonged course of rehabilitation is instituted with emphasis on strengthening the deltoid and rotator cuff muscles with the arm below the shoulder.[45,46] The scapulothoracic stabilizing muscles are strengthened as well. Patients with multidirectional instability occasionally may develop a secondary impingement syndrome. At times, a subacromial injection of a steroid preparation will provide relief sufficient for the patient to resume an exercise regimen. Activities are modified to avoid those that stress

the shoulder. A brief course of nonsteroidal, anti-inflammatory medication may be helpful, especially when a baseline joint ache results from secondary inflammation.

Imbalances in muscle coordination have been noted in studies of patients with generalized laxity,[47] and deficits in shoulder joint proprioception, possibly important in controlling the dynamic stabilizers in response to capsular or ligamentous stretch, have been noted in unstable shoulders.[48] Therapy is aimed at improving muscle tone and coordination and generally increasing the patient's functional adaptation.

SURGICAL MANAGEMENT

INDICATIONS FOR SURGERY
If the patient has prolonged symptoms that have not responded to conservative treatment, surgery is recommended. During the rehabilitation program, motivation should be carefully assessed, both to be sure the patient is mature enough to cooperate in the rehabilitation effort required postoperatively and to identify those who are manipulating their disorder for secondary gain.[4]

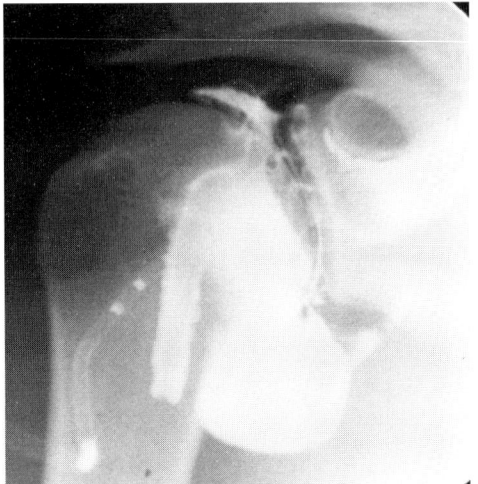 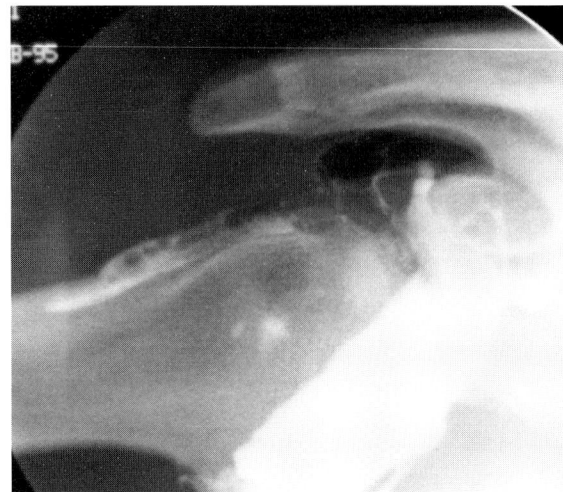

FIGURE 66
Enlarged inferior capsular pouch. **Left,** An arthrogram demonstrates capsular redundancy with an enlarged inferior pouch. **Right,** The pouch accepts the head in abduction and this patient with multidirectional instability had symptomatic inferior instability in abduction as well as a sulcus sign in adduction.

Patients with acquired instability may have developed the ability to dislocate the shoulder at will. This is especially true if certain positions will reliably result in a dislocation (eg, the humeral head falls out posteriorly whenever the arm is raised in the forward plane). Such "positional dislocators" may demonstrate this for the examiner, if requested, but otherwise do their best to avoid such positions (Fig. 65). Although "positional dislocators" can demonstrate instability on command, they do not necessarily have accompanying psychiatric disorders and are amenable to surgical correction.

These patients must be differentiated, however, from true voluntary dislocators who may have underlying psychiatric problems and often use asymmetric muscle pull to dislocate their shoulder, or even to hold it out, to great dramatic effect (Fig. 67). To complicate things further, there is a small group of patients who have developed a habitual initiation of improper muscle firing patterns, which also produce dislocations by asymmetric muscle pull. These patients can be unaware of this pattern and may be without psychiatric disturbance. Nevertheless, both groups of "muscular dislocators" are poor candidates for stabilization procedures. Those with psychiatric disturbances need counseling, and, with respect to the shoulder, skillful neglect. The group with habitually improp-

er muscle use may be successfully treated with muscle retraining and biofeedback.[49]

TECHNIQUE

The inferior capsular shift is designed to reduce capsular volume on all sides by both thickening and overlapping the capsule on the side of greatest instability and tensioning the capsule on the inferior and opposite sides (Fig. 68). For example, in a shoulder that dislocates anteriorly and inferiorly and subluxes posteriorly, an inferior capsular shift would be performed from an anterior approach. The anterior T capsulorrhaphy thickens and tightens the anterior capsule. The inferior capsular pouch is obliterated. Finally, shifting the inferior capsule anteriorly, around the humeral neck, tensions the posterior capsule. Neer named the inferior capsular shift after this novel feature, shifting the inferior capsule to tension the opposite side of the joint. Unfortunately, this has been occasionally misinterpreted, as if this were an operation primarily or exclusively on the inferior capsule.

Neer[13] referred to the gap between the supraspinatus and subscapularis as the rotator interval and called the deeper layer at the same location the "cleft" between the SGHL and the MGHL. He believed that this cleft was generally enlarged in patients with multidirectional instabil-

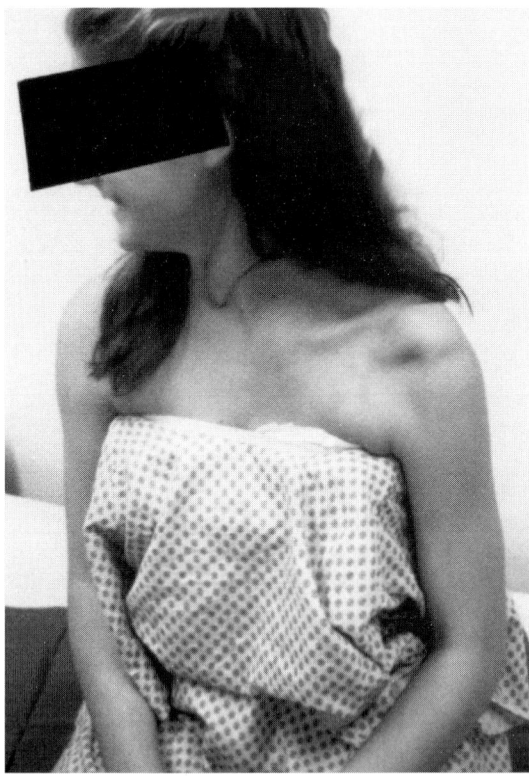

FIGURE 67
Voluntary instability. This adolescent patient is subluxing her humerus inferiorly through asymmetric muscle contraction. Although she says this is disabling, she is smiling and watching her mother's horrified reaction.

ity. Neer described closing it and drawing the superior flap tight to cause the MGHL (and the attached SGHL) "to act as a sling against inferior subluxation" (Fig. 68).[1] Thus the inferior capsular shift corrects both an enlarged inferior pouch, shown by Warner and associates[50] to be important for inferior stability in the abducted arm, and an enlarged anterosuperior (rotator interval) opening, shown in the same recent study to be important for inferior stability of the adducted arm. Neer and Foster[1] showed photographs of patients with multidirectional instability demonstrating inferior humeral subluxation in adduction and also in abduction.

The goal, to equalize tension on all sides and balance the humeral head, usually can be achieved from one surgical approach, anterior or posterior. Cooper and Brems[23] prefer to perform an anterior approach in all cases. Others have preferred to perform the approach on the side of greatest instability because this side will be best reinforced and strengthened by the overlap of flaps and the scar of the surgical approach.[7,13,22] Shoulders that dislocate both anteriorly and posteriorly should be approached from the anterior side.

Examination under anesthesia can be very helpful in confirming the components of instability. Recent biomechanical studies have contributed to the fund of knowledge regarding the static stabilizers of the glenohumeral joint and this has aided in the performance of the examination under anesthesia.[50-53] Because different portions of the capsule and ligament system are brought into play in different arm positions, the glenohumeral joint is stressed anteriorly, posteriorly, and inferiorly in adduction, 45° of abduction, 90° of abduction, and varying amounts of internal and external rotation. The direction of greatest instability usually is determined preoperatively following history taking, multiple repeat examination, plain radiography, and any additional imaging studies such as a double contrast CT arthrogram and/or MRI. It is rare to change the approach intraoperatively on the basis of the examination under anesthesia.

The surgical approaches and techniques are described above in the sections on anterior instability and posterior instability. The major modifications for the multidirectional shoulder are the extent of capsular takedown (especially how far around the humeral neck the capsule is released), the degree of overlap of the flaps, and the position and duration of postoperative immobilization. The advantage of a unified surgical approach for shoulder instability (ie, a full inferior capsular shift for multidirectional instability and a modified inferior capsular shift for unidirectional instability) is that the surgeon is not committed to any procedure from the beginning and that intermediate degrees of laxity may be dealt with precisely.

Stay sutures are placed in the capsule as it is mobilized. As the humerus is externally rotated and flexed, the capsule is incised around the neck of the humerus, extending as far posteriorly as necessary, depending on the degree of instability (Fig. 68). A finger may be placed in the inferior pouch to assess how large it is and how much redundant capsule needs to be released from the humerus prior to repair. In a shoulder with classic multidirectional instability

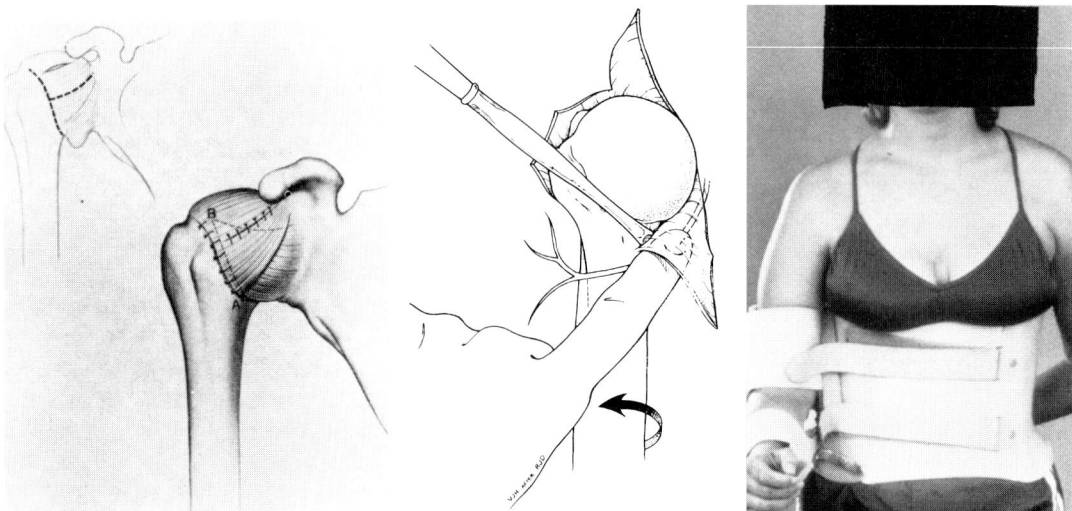

FIGURE 68

Inferior capsular shift from an anterior approach. **Left,** The capsule is reinforced and thickened anteriorly. The rotator interval and "cleft" between the superior and inferior glenohumeral ligaments is closed. Pulling the superior flap down tensions the anterosuperior capsule; pulling the inferior flap up tensions the anteroinferior capsule, and if the inferior capsule has been released around to the back, the posterior capsule is also tightened. (Reproduced with permission from Neer CS II, Foster CR: Inferior capsular shift for involuntary inferior and multidirectional instability of the shoulder: A preliminary report. *J Bone Joint Surg* 1980;62A:897-908.) **Center,** By continuing release of the capsule around the humeral neck, a precise capsulorrhaphy can be tailored to the degree of capsular laxity actually present in each case. Only the anterior capsule is freed ("modified shift") for anterior instability, while for full-blown multidirectional instability, a formal inferior capsular shift is performed by releasing around to the posterior capsule. **Right,** Brace used to immobilize patients after an inferior capsular shift. Neutral rotation avoids stretching either the anterior or posterior capsule, both of which have been tensioned by the repair. The brace sits on the iliac crests and prevents inferior sag of the arms that might stress the anterosuperior capsule.

approached from the front, the capsule is taken down all the way to the posterior capsule, which can then be tensioned as the detached inferior capsule is shifted anteriorly.

The capsule is shaped like a funnel, wider laterally. For this reason, performing the vertical limb of the T incision laterally, along the humeral neck, can most effectively shift the capsule, reducing capsular volume where the capsular circumference is largest. Also, the axillary nerve is usually close to the capsule more medially, and is more at risk with medial capsular incisions. The capsular incision is made close to the humerus, leaving a lateral remnant of tissue available for later repair. The superior cleft is also repaired to close the enlarged rotator interval.

If the glenohumeral ligament complex is detached (Broca-Perthes-Bankart lesion), it is repaired along with the capsular procedure. Ligament detachments do occur in the multidirectional shoulder, although less frequently. Anterior

glenoid bone deficiency (eg, secondary to erosion from multiple previous dislocations or from prior fracture) involving greater than 25% of the glenoid articular surface is rare, and bone grafts are almost never required in globally lax shoulders.[13]

The capsule is repaired in general with the arm in a balanced position: slight external rotation and slight flexion when anterior is the predominant direction of instability and slight extension (but still slight external rotation) when posterior is the major direction. This is modified based on the individual patient.

REHABILITATION

Patients with classic multidirectional instability are fitted with a special brace that holds the arm in a slightly abducted position with neutral rotation. The arm is immobilized in this brace for

6 weeks, allowing only gentle isometric exercises and supervised elbow range of motion during that time. At 6 weeks, the brace is discontinued and range of motion exercises are gradually introduced. At 12 weeks postoperatively, progressive strengthening is instituted on an individual basis.

An exception is often made for those patients with "bidirectional" (anterior and inferior) instability, without a significant posterior component, who are protected in a sling for 6 weeks; after 10 days, however, the arm is removed from the sling for exercises, including isometrics and external rotation to 10° and forward elevation to 90°. From 2 to 4 weeks, external rotation is increased to 30°, forward elevation is increased to 140°, and isometric strengthening is added. From 4 to 6 weeks, external rotation is increased to 40°, forward elevation is increased to approximately 160°, and resistive exercises are started. After 6 weeks, external rotation is increased to 50° and forward elevation to 180°. After 3 months, external rotation may be progressed. Strengthening begins with the arm in neutral below 90°. These are general protocols and are modified on an individual basis as indicated. The objective is to regain motion over several months, as progression that is too rapid may lead to recurrent instability. This is especially true in patients with some degree of generalized ligamentous laxity and in younger patients in late adolescence. Careful and frequent postoperative follow-up is necessary because patients who are not progressing quickly enough may need an accelerated program, while those who are regaining motion too quickly may need to be slowed down. Return to contact sports is generally restricted until after 9 to 12 months have elapsed.

RESULTS

The inferior capsular shift has become the most widely used procedure for multidirectional instability. Bony procedures as well as nonanatomic ligament suspensions and other techniques have been reported but are not used by enough centers for independent assessment of results.[2,4,54]

Since 1980, several authors have reported successful treatment of multidirectional instability with use of the inferior capsular shift.[5,9,13,23,32,54-58] In their initial report on a series of 32 patients, Neer and Foster[1] noted only one unsatisfactory result. One decade later, Neer[13] reported that an additional 100 inferior capsular shifts had similar satisfactory results.

Altchek and associates[21] reported their results following a T-plasty modification of the Bankart procedure for multidirectional instability in 42 shoulders. The patient population differed somewhat, in that 38 of the 42 cases had a Bankart lesion or detachment of the labrum and glenohumeral ligament complex. Patient satisfaction was rated excellent for 40 of the shoulders (95%). The average loss of external rotation was 5°. They noted that throwing athletes found they were unable to throw a ball with as much speed as before the operation. Additionally, seven of 42 shoulders (16%) demonstrated greater posterior instability postoperatively. There were four cases of symptomatic recurrent instability, one anterior and three posterior, while one patient required a posterior stabilization 2 years postoperatively.[21] Less favorable results were reported by Hawkins and associates[59] in a series of 31 patients followed for 2 to 5 years. Twelve (39%) went on to unsatisfactory results.

Recently Cooper and Brems[23] reviewed their series of 43 shoulders in 38 patients with a minimum 2-year follow-up after inferior capsular shift. Thirty-four shoulders (89%) rated as satisfactory with no recurrent instability. Recurrent symptomatic instability developed in four patients (11%) postoperatively. Failures and recurrences of symptomatic instability generally occurred in the early postoperative period less than 2 years after surgery.

Bigliani and associates[22] recently reported their results after inferior capsular shift for classic multidirectional instability in 52 shoulders. Thirty-six shoulders were approached from the anterior side and 16 from the posterior side. All were completely immobilized in a brace for 6 weeks postoperatively. Forty-nine shoulders were followed for from 2 to 11 years (average, 5 years). Satisfactory results were achieved in 94% of cases.

CONCLUSIONS

Controversies continue as clinical experience and basic science information are gained on multidirectional instability. Because basic science studies have shown different parts of the capsule tension in different arm positions,[50,60] it might be more physiologic to set tension in the flaps in the same fashion (eg, set the superior flap with the arm adducted and set the inferior flap with the arm abducted).[61] Given that proper repair tensioning would have to depend not only on ligament lengths at surgery but on the healing process that varies with patients (eg, some scar in and some loosen up), much remains unknown about these issues.

Several investigators have suggested a role for less than a global tensioning of the capsule—specifically, that isolated tensioning of the anterosuperior capsule and rotator interval may be helpful, especially in controlling shoulders when the predominant mode of instability is inferior.[62-64] The value of such modifications remains to be established, but initial results appear promising.

Arthroscopic techniques for capsular tensioning in multidirectional instability have been described[65] and arthroscopic laser contraction of the capsule has also been advocated.[66] However, because stiffness is a less frequent problem than recurrent instability after repairs for multidirectional instability, and because most surgeons brace or cast their patients for 6 weeks in an attempt to achieve stability, the value of minimally invasive surgery would appear less obvious.

Nonsurgical management is generally effective for most patients with multidirectional instability. If this fails, careful assessment is required to be sure the instability is the source of the patient's symptoms, to characterize the degree and direction(s) of instability, and to assess candidacy for surgical reconstruction. Once undertaken, inferior capsular shift has been an effective treatment.

REFERENCES

1. Neer CS II, Foster CR: Inferior capsular shift for involuntary inferior and multidirectional instability of the shoulder: A preliminary report. *J Bone Joint Surg* 1980;62A:897-908.

2. Bateman JE (ed): *The Shoulder and Neck,* ed 2. Philadelphia, PA, JB Lippincott, 1978, pp 475-564.

3. DePalma AF (ed): *Surgery of the Shoulder,* ed 2. Philadelphia, PA, JB Lippincott, 1973, pp 403-432.

4. Rowe CR, Pierce DS, Clark JG: Voluntary dislocation of the shoulder: A preliminary report on a clinical, electromyographic, and psychiatric study of twenty-six patients. *J Bone Joint Surg* 1973;55A:445-460.

5. Neer CS II: Involuntary inferior and multidirectional instability of the shoulder: Etiology, recognition, and treatment, in Stauffer ES (ed): American Academy of Orthopaedic Surgeons *Instructional Course Lectures XXXIV.* St. Louis, MO, CV Mosby, 1985, pp 232-238.

6. Arendt EA: Multidirectional shoulder instability. *Orthopedics* 1988;11:113-120.

7. Bigliani LU: Anterior and posterior capsular shift for multidirectional instability. *Tech Orthop* 1989;3:36-45.

8. Flatow EL: Multidirectional instability, in Kohn D (ed): *Die Schulter: Aktuelle operative Therapie.* Stuttgart, Germany, Thieme, 1992, pp 180-187.

9. Hawkins RJ, Abrams JS, Schutte J: Multidirectional instability of the shoulder: An approach to diagnosis. *Orthop Trans* 1987;11:246.

10. Hawkins RJ, Angelo RL: Glenohumeral osteoarthrosis: A late complication of the Putti-Platt repair. *J Bone Joint Surg* 1990;72A:1193-1197.

11. Hawkins RH, Hawkins RJ: Failed anterior reconstruction for shoulder instability. *J Bone Joint Surg* 1985;67B:709-714.

12. Neer CS II: Recent concepts in dislocation and subluxation, in Takagishi N (ed): *The Shoulder.* Proceedings of the Third International Conference on Surgery of the Shoulder. Tokyo, Japan, Professional Postgraduate Services, 1987, pp 7-12.

13. Neer CS II: *Shoulder Reconstruction.* Philadelphia, PA, WB Saunders, 1990, pp 273-341.

14. Norris TR, Bigliani LU: Analysis of failed repair for shoulder instability: A preliminary report, in Bateman JE, Welsh RP (eds): *Surgery of the Shoulder.* Philadelphia, PA, BC Decker, 1984, pp 111-116.

15. Rockwood CA, Gerber C: Analysis of failed surgical procedures for anterior shoulder instability. *Orthop Trans* 1985;9:48.

16. Rowe CR, Zarins B, Ciullo JV: Recurrent anterior dislocation of the shoulder after surgical repair: Apparent causes of failure and treatment. *J Bone Joint Surg* 1984;66A:159-168.

17. Steinmann SR, Flatow EL, Glasgow M, et al: Evaluation and surgical treatment of failed shoulder instability repairs. *Orthop Trans* 1992;16:727.

18. Young DC, Rockwood CA Jr: Complications of a failed Bristow procedure and their management. *J Bone Joint Surg* 1991;73A:969-981.

19. Neer CS II: *Shoulder Reconstruction.* Philadelphia, PA, WB Saunders, 1990, p 279.

20. Samilson RL, Prieto V: Dislocation arthropathy of the shoulder. *J Bone Joint Surg* 1983;65A:456-460.

21. Altchek DW, Warren RF, Ortiz G, et al: T-Plasty: A technique for treating multidirectional instability in the athlete. *Orthop Trans* 1989;13:560-561.

22. Bigliani LU, Pollock RG, Owens JM, et al: The inferior capsular shift procedure for multidirectional instability of the shoulder. *Orthop Trans* 1993;17:576.

23. Cooper RA, Brems JJ: The inferior capsular-shift procedure for multidirectional instability of the shoulder. *J Bone Joint Surg* 1992;74A:1516-1521.

24. Cordasco FA, Pollock RG, Flatow EL, et al: Management of multidirectional instability. *Oper Tech Sports Med* 1993;1:293-300.

25. Foster CR: Multidirectional instability of the shoulder in the athlete. *Clin Sports Med* 1983;2:355-368.

26. Gerber C, Ganz R: Diagnosis and causal therapy of shoulder instabilities. *Unfallchirurg* 1986;89:418-428.

27. Marberry TA: Experience with the Neer inferior capsular shift for multidirectional shoulder instability. *Orthop Trans* 1988;12:747.

28. Ozaki J: Glenohumeral movements of the involuntary inferior and multidirectional instability. *Clin Orthop* 1989;238:107-111.

29. Fu FH, Burkhead WZ Jr, Flatow EL, et al: Controversies in reconstruction of the unstable shoulder: Part 1. Mobility versus instability. *Contemp Orthop* 1993;26:301-322.

30. Fu FH, Burkhead WZ Jr, Flatow EL, et al: Controversies in reconstruction of the unstable shoulder: Part 2. Mobility versus instability. *Contemp Orthop* 1993;26:407-427.

31. Mok DW, Fogg AJ, Hokan R, et al: The diagnostic value of arthroscopy in glenohumeral instability. *J Bone Joint Surg* 1990;72B:698-700.

32. Bigliani LU, Kurzweil PR, Schwartzbach CC, et al: Inferior capsular shift procedure for anterior-inferior shoulder instability in athletes. *Am J Sports Med* 1994;22:578-584.

33. Belle RM: Collagen typing in multidirectional instability of the shoulder. *Orthop Trans* 1989;13:680-681.

34. Carter C, Sweetnam R: Recurrent dislocation of the patella and of the shoulder: Their association with familial joint laxity. *J Bone Joint Surg* 1960;42B:721-727.

35. Emery RJ, Mullaji AB: Glenohumeral joint instability in normal adolescents: Incidence and significance. *J Bone Joint Surg* 1991;73B:406-408.

36. Endo H, Takigawa T, Takata K, et al: A method of diagnosis and treatment for loose shoulder. *Cent Jpn J Orthop Surg Traumat* 1971;14:630-632.

37. Finsterbush A, Pogrund H: The hypermobility syndrome: Musculoskeletal complaints in 100 consecutive cases of generalized joint hypermobility. *Clin Orthop* 1982;168:124-127.

38. Jerosch J, Castro WH: Shoulder instability in Ehlers-Danlos Syndrome: An indication for surgical treatment? *Acta Orthopaedica Belgica* 1990;56:451-453.

39. Mallon WJ, Speer KP: Multidirectional instability: Current concepts. *J Shoulder Elbow Surg* 1995;4:54-64.

40. O'Driscoll SW, Evans DC: The incidence of contralateral shoulder instability in patients treated for recurrent anterior instability: An epidemiological investigation. *Orthop Trans* 1991;15:762.

41. Hawkins RJ, Bokor DJ: Clinical evaluation of shoulder problems, in Rockwood CA Jr, Matsen FA III (eds): *The Shoulder.* Philadelphia, PA, WB Saunders, 1990, vol 1, pp 167-171.

42. Silliman JF, Hawkins RJ: Classification and physical diagnosis of instability of the shoulder. *Clin Orthop* 1993;291:7-19.

43. Jalovaara P, Myllyla V, Paivansalo M: Autotraction stress roentgenography for demonstration anterior and inferior instability of the shoulder joint. *Clin Orthop* 1992;284:136-143.

44. Friedman RJ, Bonutti PM, Genez B, et al: Cine magnetic resonance imaging of the glenohumeral joint. Proceedings of the American Academy of Orthopaedic Surgeons 60th Annual Meeting, San Francisco, CA. Rosemont, IL, American Academy of Orthopaedic Surgeons, 1993, p 207.

45. Burkhead WZ Jr, Rockwood CA Jr: Treatment of instability of the shoulder with an exercise program. *J Bone Joint Surg* 1992;74A:890-896.

46. Rockwood CA Jr: Management of patients with multi-directional instability of the shoulder. *Orthop Trans* 1994;18:328.

47. Kronberg M, Brostrom L-A, Nemeth G: Differences in shoulder muscle activity between patients with generalized joint laxity and normal controls. *Clin Orthop* 1991;269:181-192.

48. Lephart SM, Warner JJP, Borsa PA, et al: Proprioception of the shoulder joint in healthy, unstable, and surgically repaired shoulders. *J Shoulder Elbow Surg* 1994;3:371-380.

49. Beall MS Jr, Diefenbach G, Allen A: Electromyographic biofeedback in the treatment of voluntary posterior instability of the shoulder. *Am J Sports Med* 1987;15:175-178.

50. Warner JJ, Deng XH, Warren RF, et al: Static capsuloligamentous restraints to superior-inferior translation of the glenohumeral joint. *Am J Sports Med* 1992;20:675-685.

51. Cofield RH, Nessler JP, Weinstabl R: Diagnosis of shoulder instability by examination under anesthesia. *Clin Orthop* 1993:291;45-53.

52. Harryman DT II, Sidles JA, Harris SL, et al: Laxity of the normal glenohumeral joint: A quantitative in vivo assessment. *J Shoulder Elbow Surg* 1992;1:66-76.

53. O'Brien SJ, Neves MC, Arnoczky SP, et al: The anatomy and histology of the inferior glenohumeral ligament complex of the shoulder. *Am J Sports Med* 1990;18:449-456.

54. Nobuhara K, Ikeda H: Glenoid osteotomy for loose shoulder, in Bateman JE, Welsh RP (eds): *Surgery of the Shoulder.* Philadelphia, PA, BC Decker, 1984, pp 100-103.

55. Lebar RD, Alexander AH: Multidirectional shoulder instability: Clinical results of inferior capsular shift in an active-duty population. *Am J Sports Med* 1992;20:193-198.

56. Mizuno K, Itakura Y, Muratsu H: Inferior capsular shift for inferior and multidirectional instability of the shoulder in young children: Report of two cases. *J Shoulder Elbow Surg* 1992;1:200-206.

57. Pollock RG, Owens JM, Nicholson GP, et al: Anterior inferior capsular shift procedure for anterior glenohumeral instability: Long-term results. Proceedings of the American Academy of Orthopaedic Surgeons 60th Annual Meeting, San Francisco, CA. Rosemont, IL, American Academy of Orthopaedic Surgeons, 1993, p 133.

58. Welsh RP, Trimmings N: Multidirectional instability of the shoulder. *Orthop Trans* 1987;11:231.

59. Hawkins RJ, Kunkel SS, Nayak NK: Inferior capsular shift for multidirectional instability of the shoulder: 2-5 year follow-up. *Orthop Trans* 1991;15:765.

60. Turkel SJ, Panio MW, Marshall JL, et al: Stabilizing mechanisms preventing anterior dislocation of the glenohumeral joint. *J Bone Joint Surg* 1981;63A:1208-1217.

61. Johnson DL, Warner JJP, Caborn DN, et al: The concept of a selective capsular shift for repair of anterior-inferior instability of the shoulder. Proceedings of the American Academy of Orthopaedic Surgeons 61st Annual Meeting, New Orleans, LA. Rosemont, IL, American Academy of Orthopaedic Surgeons, 1994, p 431.

62. Field LD, Warren RF, O'Brien SJ, et al: Isolated closure of rotator interval defects for shoulder instability. *J Shoulder Elbow Surg* 1995;4:S64.

63. Nobuhara K, Ikeda H: Rotator interval lesion. *Clin Orthop* 1987;223:44-50.

64. Ovesen J, Nielsen S: Experimental distal subluxation in the glenohumeral joint. *Arch Orthop Trauma Surg* 1985;104:78-81.

65. Duncan R, Savoie FH III: Arthroscopic inferior capsular shift for multidirectional instability of the shoulder: A preliminary report. *Arthroscopy* 1993;9:24-27.

66. Thabit G III: Laser-assisted capsular shift for the treatment of glenohumeral instability. *Orthopedics* 1994;3:10-12.

GLENOHUMERAL INSTABILITY IN OVERHEAD ATHLETES

JAMES E. TIBONE, MD

The overhead athlete (eg, pitchers; throwers; swimmers; volleyball, tennis, and water polo players; and javelin throwers) has unique problems about the shoulder. Overhead sports subject the shoulder to repetitive stresses, which can cause microtrauma to the static stabilizers. If the tissues do not have time to repair between stresses, permanent capsular and/or labral damage can occur, which can result in shoulder instability. The overhead athlete usually presents with shoulder pain or discomfort that affects performance rather than complaining about glenohumeral instability. In the past, the primary etiology of this shoulder pain was believed to be subacromial impingement. However, when impingement surgeries were performed on these athletes, including open or arthroscopic acromioplasties,[1-3] the results in the high-level athlete were very disappointing and did not allow the athlete to return to a competitive level. It became evident that the pain in the shoulder may not be originating primarily from subacromial impingement, but rather that this was secondary to the primary pathology, subtle glenohumeral instability.

PATHOPHYSIOLOGY

The shoulder is the most mobile joint in the body. It is unique in that it allows nonphysiologic motions such as pitching a ball while still maintaining a stable joint. Stability of the shoulder is primarily a combination of two factors. The first factor is the static stabilizers, which include the capsule and glenoid labrum. The second factor is the dynamic stabilizers, which include the rotator cuff and scapular rotators. Coordinated muscle activity of the rotator cuff and scapular rotator muscles is mandatory to maintain shoulder stability during overhead sports. If the muscles fatigue or do not fire in a proper synchronous pattern, increased stresses on the anterior capsule and labrum result. Jobe and associates[4] called this the instability continuum. The continual overhead activity that places the shoulder in maximum external rotation with 90° elevation can stretch the anterior static restraints. The dynamic stabilizers, namely the rotator cuff and scapular rotator muscles, increase their activity to compensate for this mild, clinically silent instability. The dynamic stabilizers eventually fatigue, which allows for increased instability and anterior subluxation. The anterior subluxation leads to increased translation, which causes rotator cuff "tendinitis."

This tendinitis, or rotator cuff microtearing, may be caused by glenoid impingement. Walch and associates[5] and Jobe and Sidles (unpublished data, 1992) have both reported on the intra-articular impingement between the undersurface of the rotator cuff (supraspinatus/infraspinatus) and the posterior superior labrum (Fig. 69). Elevation of the shoulder in the coronal plane with external rotation tightens the anterior capsule and ligamentous structures,[6] which causes obligate posterior humeral translation of approximately 4 mm.[7,8] When the anterior ligamentous structures are loose, this obligate posterior translation does not occur and the humeral head remains in a more

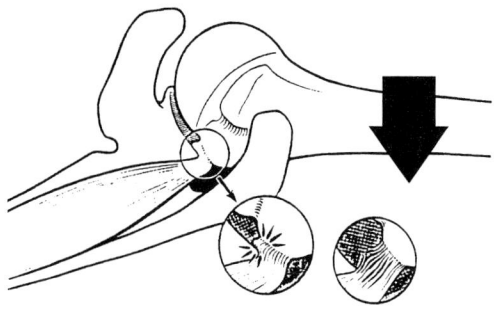

FIGURE 69

Schematic representation of posterosuperior glenoid impingement between posterior edge of glenoid and deep surface of supraspinatus and infraspinatus tendons.

anterior position. This anterior position increases contact between the undersurface of the supraspinatus and the posterior superior glenoid rim, causing further damage to the rotator cuff, with resulting pain and weakness. This weakness further aggravates the instability, resulting in a vicious cycle.

This interplay between the static and dynamic stabilizers has been confirmed in the laboratory. Electromyelography showed abnormal muscle activity in the throwing athlete with instability.[9] The activity of the subscapularis and serratus anterior muscles were markedly decreased in this group of athletes, which was thought to increase the stresses on the anterior static stabilizers.

DIAGNOSIS

The diagnosis of shoulder problems in the overhead athlete is difficult. The most important elements in the diagnosis are a comprehensive history and physical examination. Athletes usually present with pain during overhead activity. The pain may be vague and poorly localized or it may be anterior, superior, or posterior. The athlete must be asked when the pain occurs. Commonly, the pain can be localized to a specific phase of overhead activity, such as the cocking or acceleration phase of throwing. The pain may progress to activities of daily living, or may even be experienced at rest if the rotator cuff is injured. A "dead arm syndrome" is uncommon.[10] The athlete does not report that the shoulder is slipping or that it is going out of place. For example, a pitcher may report only that it takes longer for the arm to warm up, that he or she does not have control in the later innings, or that the arm does not feel as strong, or that it does not have the same endurance.

During the physical examination, the symptomatic shoulder should be compared to the asymptomatic one. Examination of the dominant shoulder of an overhead thrower is not the same as that for the nondominant shoulder, even in asymptomatic individuals. The dominant shoulder of the thrower usually has increased external rotation, especially in the abducted position, with a concomitant decrease in internal rotation. During stability testing, the dominant shoulder will have increased transla-

tion compared to the nondominant shoulder. An apprehension test, or a "crank maneuver," usually does not cause apprehension, but it can cause pain. Jobe and associates[4] and Kvitne and Jobe[11] have described a relocation test to differentiate pain with the crank maneuver. The athlete is supine with the involved shoulder at the edge of the examining table and the shoulder is placed in 90° abduction with full external rotation. The examiner applies an anterior force to the humeral head, which will cause pain but not apprehension in the athlete with mild anterior instability. The same maneuver is performed with a posteriorly directed force on the humeral head (Fig. 70). "Relocating the head" should eliminate the pain. The pain relieved by this maneuver is believed to be caused by impingement of the undersurface of the supraspinatus on the superior glenoid rim. Posteriorly directed pressure on the humeral head restores the space between the rotator cuff and the glenoid rim, thereby relieving the pain. If the pain is not caused by instability with glenoid impingement, the relocation maneuver should not eliminate the pain.

The classic impingement signs of Neer[12] and Hawkins and Kennedy[13] are usually positive in the athlete with shoulder pain. Besides subacromial impingement, a positive sign can be the result of inflammation of the rotator cuff tendons and bursa. The classic impingement maneuver in studies using cadavers shows that there can be glenoid impingement of the undersurface of the rotator cuff (CM Jobe, personal communication).

Glenoid translation is measured comparing one shoulder to the other. Translation that is measured in the neutral position, however, does not test the static stabilizers of the shoulder. The shoulder should be placed in different positions of external rotation to test the competency of the glenohumeral ligaments. The most important stabilizing structure for the overhead athlete, the anterior band of the inferior glenohumeral ligament,[6,14] becomes taut in the cocking position of throwing (90° abduction, 90° external rotation). The athlete should be examined in 90° of abduction with different degrees of external rotation to determine when the glenohumeral ligaments become tight. The results should be compared to the unaffected shoulder. However, a slight amount of asymmetry with these maneuvers would not be unexpected.

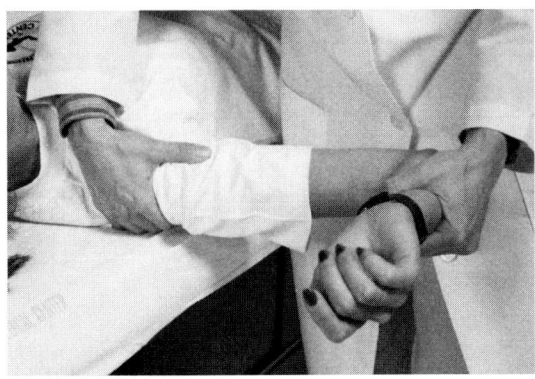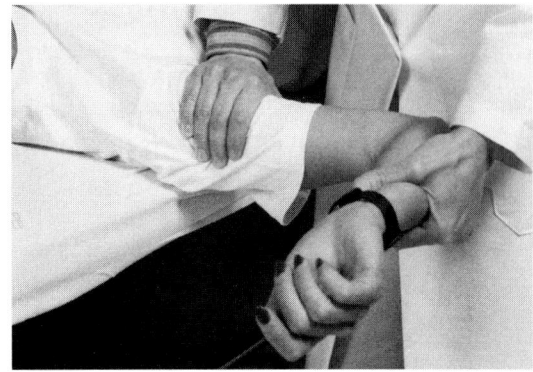

FIGURE 70
Left, Apprehension test. Arm is placed in abducted and externally rotated position, with forward stress applied to humeral head. Pain is felt by patient who had instability, and apprehension is felt by patient who has dislocation. **Right,** Relocation test. Arm is placed in same position as in apprehension test, and posterior stress is applied to humeral head. Relief from pain and possibility relocation of humeral head are indicative of anterior instability.

A sulcus sign, performed by applying downward pressure on the arm while the arm is at the side, is useful to evaluate inferior laxity. The examination should also include an evaluation for scapula asymmetry and a slight scapular lag with elevation. If the athlete is examined during throwing, a drop in the elbow during cocking and increased trunk motion with increased lumbar lordosis may be evident. With poor trunk mechanics, the additional stress placed on the shoulder can lead to the beginning of the instability complex.

DIAGNOSTIC STUDIES

Routine radiographic examination is mandatory in any patient with shoulder pain. However, in evaluating the young overhead athlete, radiographs do not usually give any additional information. Overhead athletes with instability secondary to repetitive microtrauma do not usually have a Hill-Sachs deformity of the posterior humeral head because they have never had a true dislocation. For the same reason, there is usually no bony Bankart lesion on the anterior inferior rim. Additional studies, such as CT arthrograms and MRIs, are usually not helpful. Data from these studies are usually confusing and add little to making the definitive diagnosis. The cost-effec-

tiveness of CT and MRI studies in a young athletic population must be questioned.

An overhead athlete with shoulder pain that does not respond to a conservative exercise program, should be examined under anesthesia and with diagnostic arthroscopy to confirm the diagnosis. Findings at arthroscopy can be subtle. A classic Bankart lesion and/or Hill-Sachs lesion is absent in overhead athletes. The findings at arthroscopy that suggest anterior instability include labral separation and damage, absent or stretched ligaments, a positive "drive-through sign," ligaments that do not tighten with external rotation of the shoulder, posterior humeral head chondromalacia, and undersurface fraying of the supraspinatus that corresponds to an area of impingement on the posterior superior glenoid when the arm is placed in the cocking position of throwing.[5,11,15,16]

CLASSIFICATION

The overhead athlete with shoulder pain can usually be classified into one of four groups based on the history, physical examination, and arthroscopic findings.[4] Group I patients have shoulder pain caused by subacromial impingement but have no shoulder instability. On examination, these athletes have classic impingement signs.

They may also have pain in the apprehensive position; however, pain is not relieved by a relocation test. Translation is not increased during stability testing and arthroscopic evaluation shows a normal labrum and normal glenohumeral ligaments. Rotator cuff fraying may be present; however, the sine qua non is a subacromial space that is inflamed and fibrotic.

Group II patients have chronic repetitive microtrauma causing primary instability and secondary impingement. The secondary impingement in these cases is usually glenoid impingement rather than subacromial impingement. On examination, the athletes have positive impingement signs and a positive relocation test. Examination demonstrates increased translation and the arthroscopic findings show subtle signs of instability, which may include rotator cuff fraying, as mentioned above. This is the largest group of overhead athletes with shoulder pain.

Group III patients have ligamentous laxity that causes shoulder instability. They also develop a secondary impingement, which again is usually glenoid in nature but may have a subacromial component. On examination, they exhibit obvious signs of hyperelasticity, including recurvatum of the elbows and the ability to touch the thumb to the forearm. Impingement testing elicits pain and the relocation test is positive. Examination of the shoulder reveals large translation in all directions, which usually is also present in the asymptomatic shoulder. Also, the finding during arthroscopic evaluation may be minimal, but occasionally there is undersurface rotator cuff fraying and/or poorly developed glenohumeral ligaments. Swimmers are commonly found in this group.

Group IV patients have typical traumatic anterior instability without impingement. The history includes a significant traumatic event that produces an episode of glenohumeral instability. In baseball, the most common etiology is sliding into a base. Examination does not show impingement. Group IV is the only group that has apprehension in addition to pain with a "crank test." Symptoms are relieved with a relocation maneuver. Examination under anesthesia reveals translations greater than usual in the normal shoulder and anterior ligaments that do not tighten with external rotation. These athletes will have a classic Bankart lesion and Hill-Sachs deformity.

TREATMENT

CONSERVATIVE MANAGEMENT

Most overhead athletes respond to a nonsurgical program to relieve shoulder pain. The static stabilizers must be rested. This does not mean that the shoulder should be placed in a sling or shoulder immobilizer. The athlete should rest the shoulder from overhead activities. Nonsteroidal anti-inflammatory medications, used in maximum doses for 7 to 10 days, should be taken to reduce the inflammation in the shoulder before an exercise program is started. Cortisone injections can also be used to reduce the inflammation in the tendons. This steroid does not cause any untoward effects as long as the athlete does not compete immediately after the injection. Most athletes respond to one injection, but up to three may be given over a 6-month period. The judicious use of ice in the early stages has been shown to reduce swelling.

The major component of conservative care is an exercise program to strengthen the dynamic stabilizers, which include the rotator cuff and scapula rotator muscles, and to re-establish scapuloglenoid rhythm. An efficient, effective core exercise program has been developed to stress these shoulder muscles.[17-19] The program includes elevation in the scapular plane with the thumbs up, shoulder flexion, a press-up performed on a chair, horizontal abduction with the shoulder externally rotated, horizontal rowing, and a push-up plus. It is important that the athlete with anterior instability perform the exercises in the scapular plane and avoid performing the exercises in the coronal plane of the body. No stretching exercises for the anterior capsule are performed. The posterior capsule is usually tight, which can aggravate anterior instability. Towel stretches can easily be used to stretch the posterior capsule.

A conservative program is continued for at least 6 months before surgical intervention is considered. Occasionally, diagnostic arthroscopy may be needed before this time to reassure the athlete and obtain an exact diagnosis.

SURGICAL TREATMENT

If the overhead athlete has not responded to 6 months of conservative care and does not wish to limit athletic activity, surgical treatment can be considered. Diagnostic arthroscopy is always performed prior to surgery to obtain an exact diagnosis. A diagnostic arthroscopy does not preclude standard open shoulder surgery under the same anesthetic. The choice of anesthesia may be general or interscalene block; the latter achieves excellent muscle relaxation while avoiding some of the complications of general anesthesia. The occasional athlete with pure subacromial impingement (group I) is treated with a conventional acromioplasty, coracoacromial ligament excision, and bursectomy. Athletes in groups II, III, and IV, whose major pathology is anterior instability, are treated with an anterior capsular repair. A group IV patient with pure traumatic anterior instability may forego the conservative regimen because of the high recurrence rate and undergo a surgical repair that will allow a high-level athlete to maintain full function of the shoulder and lose a minimal amount of competitive time.

A modification of the Bankart repair, an anterior capsulolabral reconstruction,[11,16,20] developed by Jobe, is a successful treatment option for the overhead athlete. There are several principles with this procedure: no muscles are detached, excessive tightening of the glenohumeral capsule is avoided, the capsule at the site of instability (namely, the glenoid rim) is reinforced, rehabilitation is immediate, and a full range of motion necessary for maximum function is obtained. During this procedure, the subscapularis muscle is split rather than detached. The anterior capsule is tightened and overlapped in a superior-inferior direction; medial-lateral shortening of the capsule is avoided. Mitek suture anchors allow the procedure to be performed easily through this more limited exposure, while avoiding injury to the articular cartilage.

SURGICAL TECHNIQUE

The patient is placed in a supine position with the arm away from the side, supported by an arm board or Parker table. A standard anterior skin incision in the lines of tension and a deltopectoral approach is performed to the level of the subscapularis. With the shoulder in external rotation, the exposed subscapularis is split in the direction of its fibers at the junction of the upper two thirds of the tendon with the lower one third (Fig. 71). The subscapularis muscle is dissected free from the underlying capsule. It is usually easier to

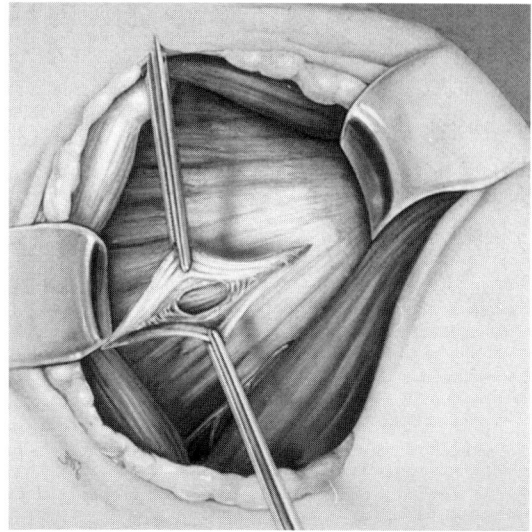

FIGURE 71
Subscapularis muscle split at junction of upper two thirds and lower one third.

begin medially where the muscle can be easily separated from the capsule. Laterally, the tendon and capsule become confluent and are more difficult to separate. In this area, the dissection must be done sharply. Once the capsule and subscapularis muscle have been separated, a bent Gelpi retractor separates the subscapularis, and a pitchfork retractor can be placed underneath the subscapularis muscle on the glenoid neck (Fig. 72). The capsule is then also divided horizontally from lateral to medial, to about the 3 o'clock position on the glenoid. If the capsular cut is made too inferior on the glenoid, the anterior band of the inferior glenohumeral ligament will be divided. The humeral head retractor is then placed across the glenohumeral joint. A Bankart lesion is usually not present, so care must be taken not to cut the anterior glenoid labrum. The inner synovial layer of the capsule is freed from the labrum and the capsule and periosteum are elevated from the anterior scapular neck just medial to the intact labrum. A #2 Mitek drill bit is used to make three drill holes along the anterior glenoid margin, just medial to the articular edge and labrum. These drill holes are usually made at the 5, 4, and 3 o'clock positions for a right shoulder (Fig. 73). The #2 Mitek double-prong anchor is then inserted into each hole with its attached #2 Ethibond suture. The

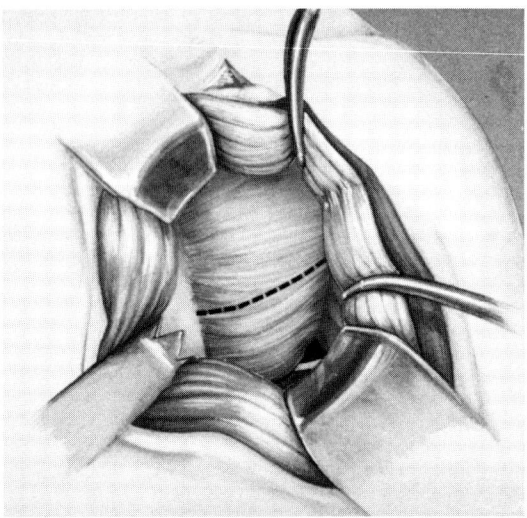

FIGURE 72
Glenohumeral joint capsule exposure. Dotted line indicates site of capsulotomy.

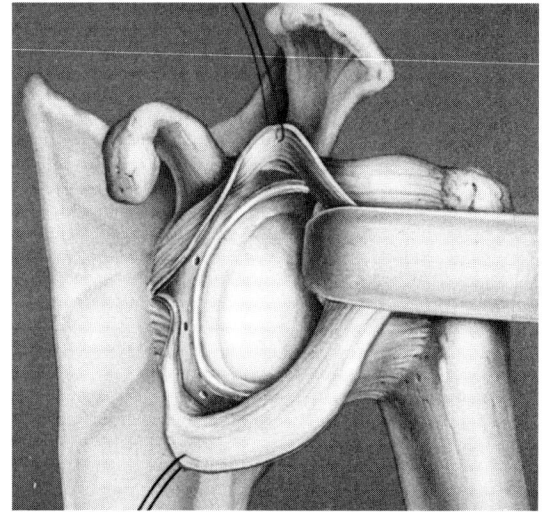

FIGURE 73
Drill holes located along anterior glenoid rim.

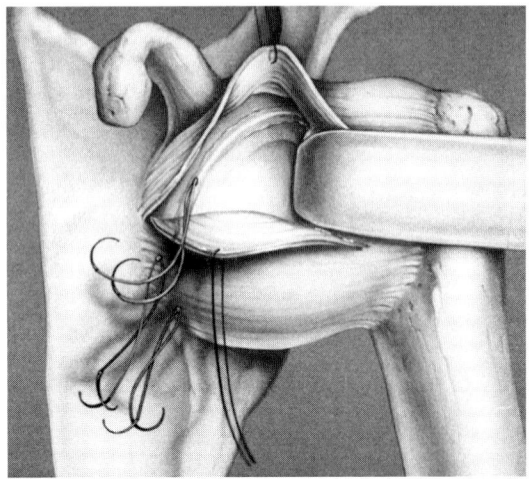

FIGURE 74
Inferior capsular flap shifted superiorly and anchored into position.

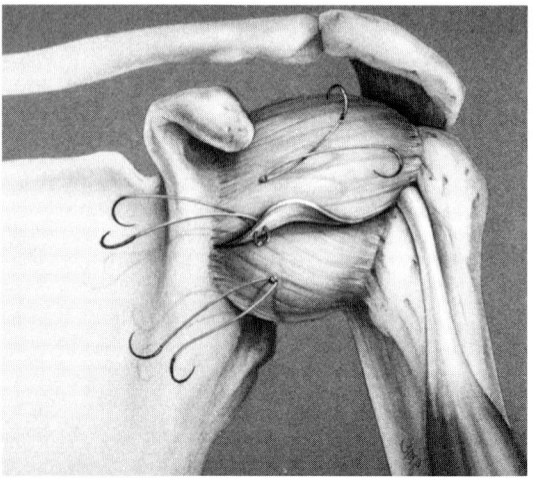

FIGURE 75
Superior capsular flap shifted inferiorly, overlying the inferior flap.

inferior capsular flap is advanced superiorly and secured to the glenoid rim with the Ethibond sutures (Fig. 74). Care must be taken to place these sutures at the medial edge of the capsule. Lateral placement of these sutures causes exces-

sive capsular tightening and postoperative restriction of motion. The superior capsular flap is then brought inferiorly over the inferior capsular flap and sutured in position (Fig. 75). In the overhead athlete, the shoulder should be able to be positioned in 90° abduction and at least 75° of external rotation without disrupting the repair. The remaining split in the capsule is closed, along with the split in the subscapularis muscle.

POSTOPERATIVE REHABILITATION

The overhead athlete is placed in a shoulder orthosis that maintains the shoulder in 90° elevation in the plane of the scapula and 45° external rotation (Fig. 76). This position prevents inferior capsular scarring, which allows easier rehabilitation and earlier return of full range of motion. The orthosis is worn at all times during the first 2 weeks, except during the physical therapy program, which is started on the first day postoperatively.

Passive range of motion is started immediately in the scapular plane, with external rotation performed within the safe zone, determined at the time of surgery. Exercises are started at the side and progressed to the prone and side-lying positions. By 3 months, the athlete has full range of motion, except for some minor restriction of full external rotation. Sports can be started at 6 months and a progressive throwing program can be started at that time. It will take a thrower 12 months to return to a competitive status.

Seventy-five overhead athletes evaluated with a minimum of 28 months follow-up after an anterior capsulolabral reconstruction reported an average loss of external rotation in the throwing position of 2°.[21] Results were excellent in 77%, good in 15%, fair in 3%, and poor in 5%. Excellent results were reported in six of 13 professional pitchers and seven of seven collegiate pitchers. Fifteen of 20 professional baseball players returned to the same level of competition. Overall in the series, 77% of athletes returned to the same competitive level.

ARTHROSCOPIC STABILIZATION

Arthroscopic procedures have become increasingly popular in recent years. It is enticing to use such a procedure on an athlete to avoid the morbidity of an open surgery. At present, however, arthroscopic procedures are not recommended in

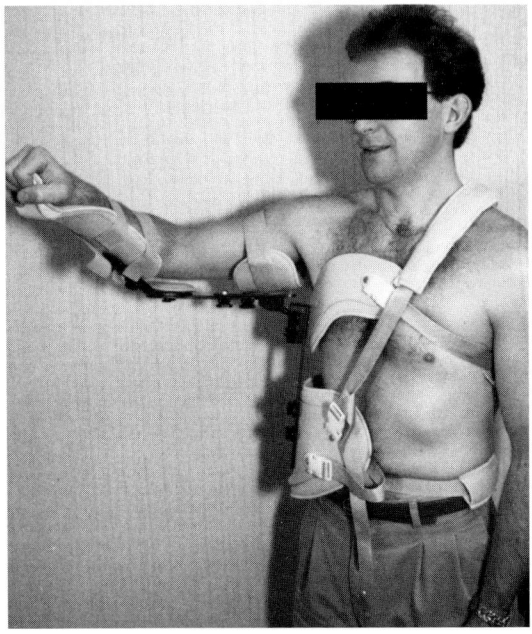

FIGURE 76
Postoperative orthosis.

the overhead athlete, especially because these athletes do not have a true Bankart lesion. These athletes often have significant capsular stretching, which is very difficult to correct arthroscopically. In addition, the high-level athlete cannot afford the higher failure rate, which has been documented with arthroscopic procedures.[22,23] At the present time, arthroscopic stabilization may have a role in first-time traumatic dislocation (group IV patients), but this is not the usual situation in the overhead athlete.[24]

REFERENCES

1. Tibone JE, Elrod B, Jobe FW, et al: Surgical treatment of tears of the rotator cuff in athletes. *J Bone Joint Surg* 1986;68A:887-891.

2. Tibone JE, Jobe FW, Kerlan RK, et al: Shoulder impingement syndrome in athletes treated by an anterior acromioplasty. *Clin Orthop* 1985;198:134-140.

3. Fly WR, Tibone JE, Glousman, RE: Arthroscopic subacromial decompression in athletes less than 40 years old. *Orthop Trans* 1990;14:250-251.

4. Jobe FW, Kvitne RS, Giangarra CE: Shoulder pain in the overhand or throwing athlete: The relationship of anterior instability and rotator cuff impingement. *Orthop Rev* 1989;18:963-975.

5. Walch G, Bioleau P, Noel E, et al: Impingement of the deep surface of the supraspinatus tendon on the posterosuperior glenoid rim: An arthroscopic study. *J Shoulder Elbow Surg* 1992; 1:238-245.

6. Turkel SJ, Panio MW, Marshall JL, et al: Stabilizing mechanisms preventing anterior dislocation of the glenohumeral joint. *J Bone Joint Surg* 1981;63A:1208-1217.

7. Harryman DT II, Sidles JA, Clark JM, et al: Translation of the humeral head on the glenoid with passive glenohumeral motion. *J Bone Joint Surg* 1990;72A:1334-1343.

8. Howell SM, Galinat BJ, Renzi AJ, et al: Normal and abnormal mechanics of the glenohumeral joint in the horizontal plane. *J Bone Joint Surg* 1988;70A:227-232.

9. Glousman R, Jobe F, Tibone J, et al: Dynamic electromyographic analysis of the throwing shoulder with glenohumeral instability. *J Bone Joint Surg* 1988;70A:220-226.

10. Rowe CR: Recurrent transient anterior subluxation of the shoulder: The "dead-arm syndrome." *Clin Orthop* 1987;223:11-19.

11. Kvitne RS, Jobe FW: The diagnosis and treatment of anterior instability in the throwing athlete. *Clin Orthop* 1993;291:107-123.

12. Neer CS II: Anterior acromioplasty for the chronic impingement syndrome in the shoulder: A preliminary report. *J Bone Joint Surg* 1972;54A:41-50.

13. Hawkins RJ, Kennedy JC: Impingement syndromes in athletes. *Am J Sports Med* 1980;8:151-158.

14. Cain PR, Mutschler TA, Fu FH, et al: Anterior stability of the glenohumeral joint: A dynamic model. *Am J Sports Med* 1987;15:144-148.

15. McGlynn FJ, Caspari RB: Arthroscopic findings in the subluxating shoulder. *Clin Orthop* 1984;183:173-178.

16. Jobe FW, Giangarra CE, Kvitne RS, et al: Anterior capsulolabral reconstruction of the shoulder in athletes in overhand sports. *Am J Sports Med* 1991;19:428-434.

17. Townsend H, Jobe FW, Pink M, et al: Electromyographic analysis of the glenohumeral muscles during a baseball rehabilitation program. *Am J Sports Med* 1991;19:264-272.

18. Moseley JB Jr, Jobe FW, Pink M, et al: EMG analysis of the scapular muscles during a shoulder rehabilitation program. *Am J Sports Med* 1992;20:128-134.

19. Bradley JP, Tibone JE: Electromyographic analysis of muscle action about the shoulder. *Clin Sports Med* 1991;10:789-805.

20. Jobe FW, Glousman RE: Anterior capsulolabral reconstruction. *Tech Orthop* 1989;3:29-35.

21. Rubenstein DL, Jobe FW, Glousman RE, et al: Anterior capsulolabral reconstruction of the shoulder in athletes. *J Shoulder Elbow Surg* 1992;1:229-237.

22. Grana WA, Buckley PD, Yates CK: Arthroscopic Bankart suture repair. *Am J Sports Med* 1993;21:348-353.

23. Hawkins RB: Arthroscopic stapling repair for shoulder instability: A retrospective study of 50 cases. *Arthroscopy* 1989;5:122-128.

24. Arciero RA, Wheeler JH, Ryan JB, et al: Arthroscopic Bankart repair versus nonoperative treatment for acute, initial anterior shoulder dislocations. *Am J Sports Med* 1994;22:589-594.

GLENOHUMERAL INSTABILITY REPAIRS: COMPLICATIONS AND FAILURES

LOUIS U. BIGLIANI, MD

Surgical treatment of recurrent shoulder instability is well established and most patients undergoing surgical repair have a successful result. Through the years, our perspective and understanding of glenohumeral instability has evolved, and recently there have been several reports describing failed instability repairs.[1-10] In the past, glenohumeral instability was usually considered as primarily traumatic anterior dislocation. However, we have come to appreciate more subtle instability, such as subluxation, as well as posterior and multidirectional instability.

Most unsuccessful repairs are secondary to either an incorrect diagnosis, improper surgical technique, or inappropriate rehabilitation. Lack of patient cooperation can also be a consideration in failure, especially if the patient is a voluntary dislocator. Several factors have been associated with failure of instability repairs. However, the two most common factors associated with a failed instability repair are a persistent labral avulsion (Bankart, Perthes, Broca lesion) and excessive capsular laxity (Fig. 77). Both of these pathologic abnormalities involve the IGHL, which is the most important static restraint against anterior and anterior-inferior instability. One of the primary goals of any anterior instability repair should be to evaluate the integrity of this ligament and cor-

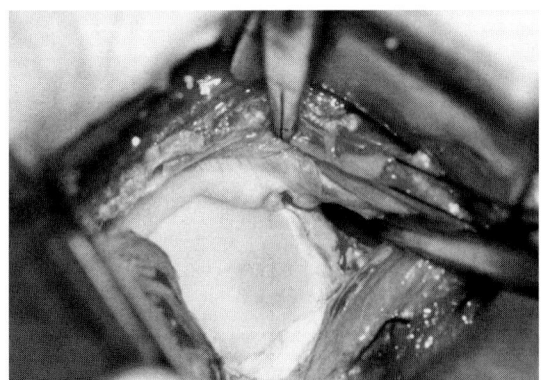
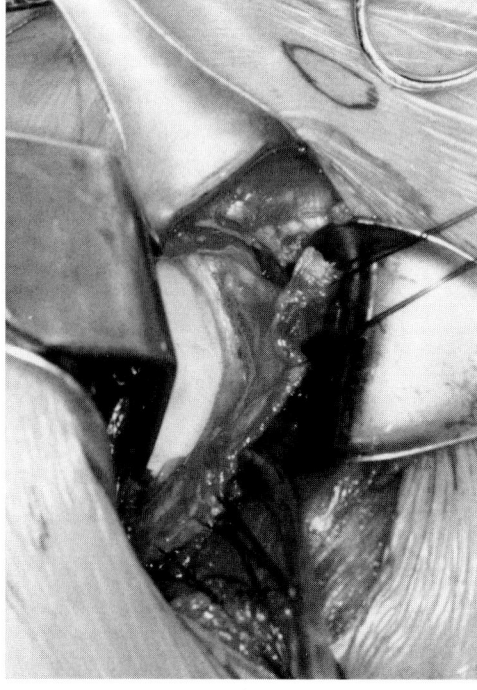

FIGURE 77

Inferior glenohumeral pathology. **Left,** A persistent labral avulsion and a Bankart lesion in a patient with recurrent anterior instability following an extra-articular repair. **Right,** Persistent excessive capsular laxity present in patient with recurrent anterior-inferior instability following an extra-articular extracapsular repair.

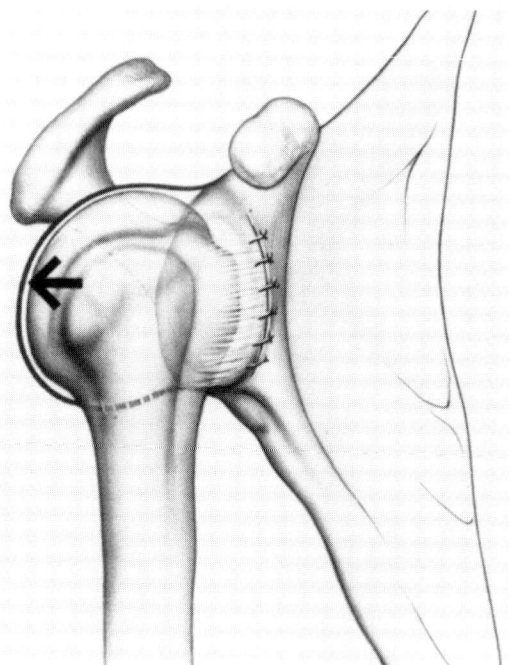

FIGURE 78

Soft-tissue procedures excessively limit external rotation and subluxate and dislocate the shoulder out in the opposite direction.

rect the deficiencies that are found. Therefore, surgical procedures that deal with extracapsular repairs cannot adequately evaluate the IGHL and correct capsular avulsion or excessive capsular laxity and should be avoided.

The IGHL attaches to most of the anterior and inferior aspect of the glenoid rim via the labrum. If the labrum is detached from the bone or if the capsule is torn from the labrum, the ability of the IGHL to act as a static restraint is compromised. Several series have reported a persistent labral detachment as an etiologic factor in failed instability repairs (Fig. 78, *left*).[1,3,4]

Excessive capsular laxity, as seen in multidirectional instability, can pose a significant surgical challenge because it is important to decrease the volume of the joint while tightening the capsule to the proper tension in an anterior, inferior, and posterior direction. The standard repairs that deal only with unidirectional instability—such as subscapularis transfer (Magnuson-Stack), subscapularis and capsular shortening (Putti-Platt), and a coracoid transfer (Bristow Latarjet procedure)—

may tighten the shoulder on one side anteriorly and subluxate the humeral head posteriorly, leading to degenerative arthritis (Fig. 78). It is important to achieve proper tissue tensioning, especially with capsular laxity, because there is a greater tendency to subluxate in the opposite direction.

Recently, several reports in the literature have focused attention on the problems with anterior instability procedures that have been made too tight. Lusardi and associates[10] reported on 20 shoulders following anterior capsulorrhaphies, the most common of which was a Magnuson-Stack procedure. There was severe loss of external rotation in all patients with 17 shoulders having pain and 16 shoulders having mild to severe glenohumeral arthrosis (Fig. 79). In addition, seven shoulders had posterior subluxation or dislocation of the humeral head. Hawkins and Angelo[2] reported severe glenohumeral arthrosis with substantial loss of external rotation following an anterior Putti-Platt procedure. Also, Bigliani and associates reported on 17 patients having severe osteoarthritis requiring prosthetic replacement. Fourteen of these patients had various soft-tissue procedures including five Putti-Platt and three Magnuson-Stack procedures. These authors recommended avoiding procedures such as the Putti-Platt and Magnuson-Stack that severely limit external rotation.

The use of hardware during an instability repair can lead to failure. Hardware can be incorrectly placed, become painful, loosen, or migrate into the glenohumeral joint (Fig. 80). Zuckerman and Matsen[6] reported a series of 37 patients who had significant complications following placement of hardware during instability repairs. Twenty-one had problems related to the use of screws to fix a coracoid transfer, while 17 had problems with staples. Thirty-four patients required a second procedure and 14 patients (41%) had significant articular surface damage. O'Driscoll and Evans[9] reported on 204 patients who had open staple capsulorrhaphies by several different surgeons. There was high percentage of postoperative instability, with 22% of shoulders having recurrent dislocations or subluxations. Twenty-four patients (12%) had problems specifically with the staple loosening, migrating, or penetrating the articular surface. Overall, 51% of patients had pain and 50% thought the shoulder was not normal. Young and Rockwood[5] reported on 40 shoulders that failed following a Bristow

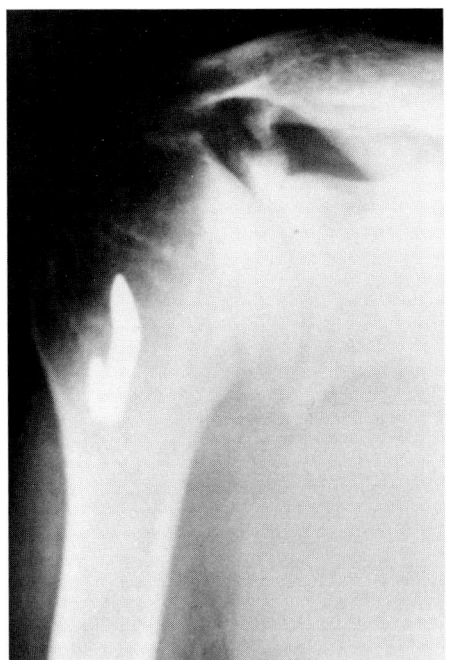
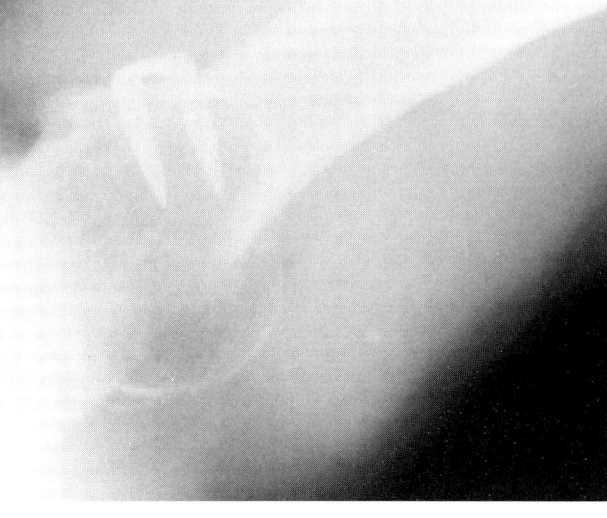

FIGURE 79
Arthritis following a subscapularis transfer. This 53-year-old patient developed progressive arthritis following a subscapularis transfer (Magnuson-Stack procedure) in which external rotation was never regained. **Left,** Anteroposterior radiographs show joint space narrowing, osteophyte formation and sclerosis. **Right,** Axillary radiograph showing posterior subluxation.

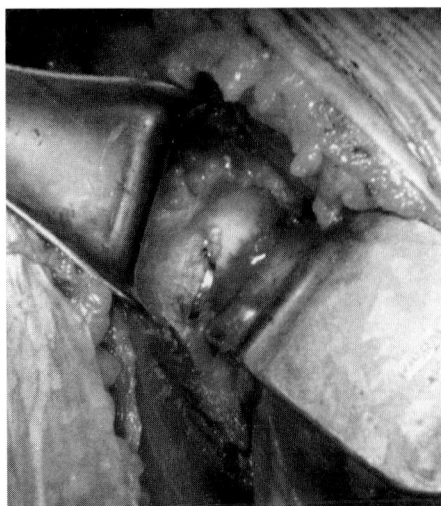
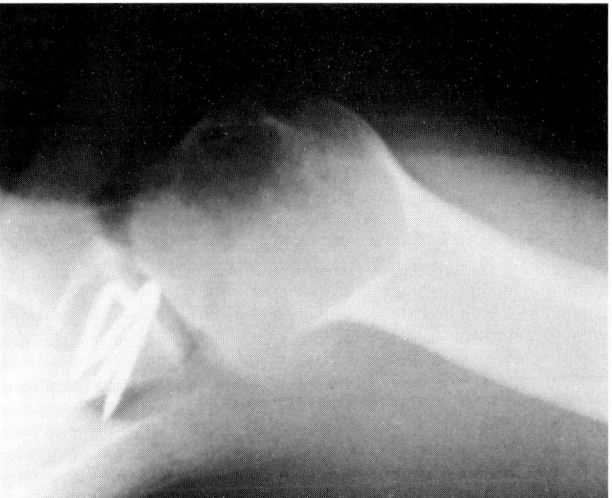

FIGURE 80
A 26-year-old male patient having articular cartilage damage following a staple capsulorrhaphy. **Left,** Surgical photograph showing two staples in the glenoid. **Right,** Axillary radiographs showing the staple in the glenoid and degenerative changes in the humeral head.

procedure (Fig. 81). In addition to loosening of the screw fixation, the other complications involved with the index Bristow procedure included recurrent painful shoulder instability, injury to the articular cartilage, failure of the coracoid bone block to unite with the glenoid, neurovascular injury, and posterior instability. Hovelius and associates[11] reported on a series of 112 patients who had the Bristow Latarjet procedure, in which there was a failure rate of 13%, consisting of six patients who had redislocations and seven who had subluxation. Technical errors were believed to be the most important factor associated with failure. The investigator thought that a bony or fibrous union must be present and the bone block should be placed inferior to the glenoid equator less than 1 cm medial to the glenoid rim. Recently, there has been less enthusiasm for the Bristow Latarjet procedure as the primary procedure in the treatment of anterior glenohumeral instability unless there is a significant bony deficiency of the anterior glenoid rim.

Neurovascular injuries can also occur secondary to an anterior instability repair. Injury to the axillary artery is uncommon but is a potentially devastating complication requiring immediate attention. Injuries to the brachial plexus as well as various individual nerves including the axillary musculocutaneous and suprascapular nerve are more common. The axillary nerve is especially vulnerable as it courses on the inferior aspect of the capsule of the glenohumeral joint, an area that is often dissected and mobilized in various types of capsular repairs. The axillary nerve should always be adequately identified during an inferior dissection. The musculocutaneous nerve also can be injured easily. The nerve lies just medial and inferior to the coracoid process, an area where retractors are often placed to gain exposure. The nerve can be injured when the tip of the coracoid and adjoining muscles are detached, mobilized, and transferred in a Bristow Latarjet procedure. It was long believed that the musculocutaneous nerve entered the coracobrachialis 5 cm or more from the tip of the coracoid. Flatow and associates[12] reported that in 29% of 93 cadaveric shoulders, the nerve penetrated the coracobrachialis less than 5 cm from the tip and as close as 3 cm. Often there were small twigs more proximal to the main nerve trunk. Injury to the suprascapular nerve is quite rare but can occur in posterior instability procedures and also with either open or arthroscopic anterior procedures that use transglenoid sutures. Richards and associates[13] reported on eight patients who had iatrogenic injuries to the various elements of the brachial plexus during a Magnuson-Stack or Putti-Platt procedure. Six patients had complete lesions of the musculocutaneous nerve, two had complete lesions of the axillary nerve, and two had lacerations of the axillary artery. The authors concluded that incomplete lesions can be followed if they show progressive recovery, and lesions that either fail to recover or recover incompletely should be explored at 3 months. Complete lesions should be explored at an earlier date and the appropriate repair performed. Other less common factors associated with failure are misdiagnosis, infection, scarring of the subscapularis and glenoid fracture, a large Hill-Sachs lesion, and inappropriate rehabilitation.

Arthroscopy has become a popular diagnostic and therapeutic procedure in the treatment of anterior instability. The specific problems associated with arthroscopy are discussed above under *Arthroscopic Bankart Repair*.

EVALUATION

A thorough evaluation of the patient with failed instability is essential. This is often difficult because the patient may have significant pain, stiffness, and instability. A detailed history is helpful. In the absence of complete dislocation the patient may report episodes of locking, catching, slipping, or even neurologic symptoms extending down the arm. A copy of the surgical report of the previous repair or repairs should be obtained, and the patient should be asked about length of immobilization and rehabilitation following the previous procedure. If possible, the patient should be assessed for anterior, inferior, and posterior instability. However, pain may preclude a reasonable examination. It is very useful to evaluate these patients under anesthesia when there is adequate relaxation and relief of pain. Norris[14] has also described a technique of using a C-arm to image the shoulder while doing the evaluation. This procedure may help to determine whether there is excessive motion of the head past the glenoid rim, which is often difficult to determine

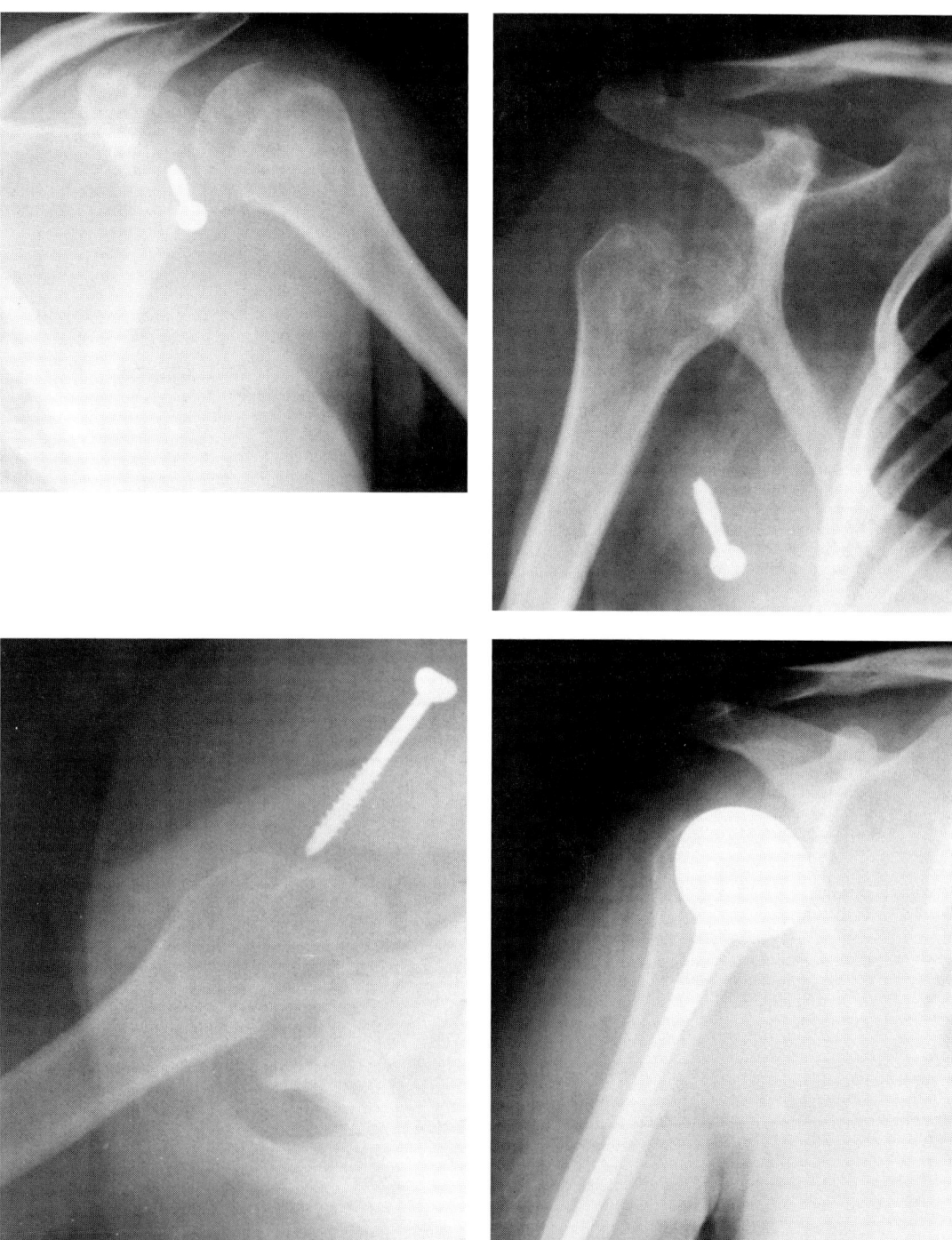

FIGURE 81

A 22-year-old female with resection of the humeral head following a Bristow procedure. **Top left,** Anteroposterior radiograph of the shoulder following a Bristow procedure. **Top right,** Anteroposterior radiograph showing a loose screw inferiorly with severe degeneration of the humeral head. **Bottom left,** Axillary radiograph showing complete destruction of the humeral head. **Bottom right,** Modular hemiarthroplasty performed to correct the arthritis of the glenohumeral joint.

objectively and which usually involves a subjective evaluation without the use of radiographic enhancement.

A patient should have a full radiologic evaluation, including an anteroposterior view of the shoulder in neutral, internal, and external rotation, a lateral view in the scapular plane, and an axillary view. The axillary view is essential to evaluate the anterior and posterior glenoid and the relationship between the humeral head and the glenoid surface. Arthritic changes are often seen on the axillary view and it is the best way to evaluate posterior wear and subluxation (Fig 80, *right*). Imaging may also be indicated to evaluate articular surfaces and direction of instability. In the past, CT arthrograms have been very helpful to evaluate the presence of any lesions of the capsule, labrum, or cartilage. MRI techniques also have been developed into useful tests for instability. If there is still significant confusion, then arthroscopy is an excellent way to evaluate the articular surfaces, labrum, and capsule prior to performing an open repair.

SURGICAL TECHNIQUE

Overall, the principles of re-repair following failed instability surgery should be to correct the persistent pathology and to restore normal anatomy. The approach should be from the side of the greatest instability or contracture. Often, the persistent pathology with extracapsular anterior repairs is often either a Bankart lesion or excessive capsular laxity. Either of these can be dealt with by performing the appropriate capsulorrhaphy procedure and correcting the subscapularis muscle and tendon to the most anatomic position. Rowe and associates[4] reported a persistent Bankart lesion or excessive capsular laxity in more than 80% of the patients treated surgically for anterior shoulder instability. The success rate was encouraging, with 22 of 24 shoulders followed for longer than 2 years having a satisfactory result with another reconstructive capsulorrhaphy. Patients with excessive inferior capsular laxity can have residual inferior laxity if an anterior repair is made too tight across the anterior aspect

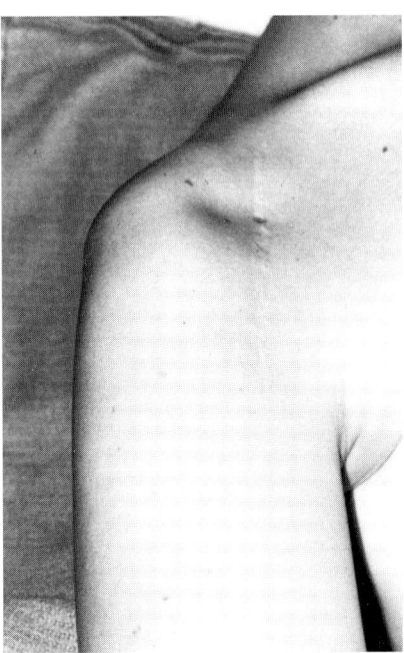 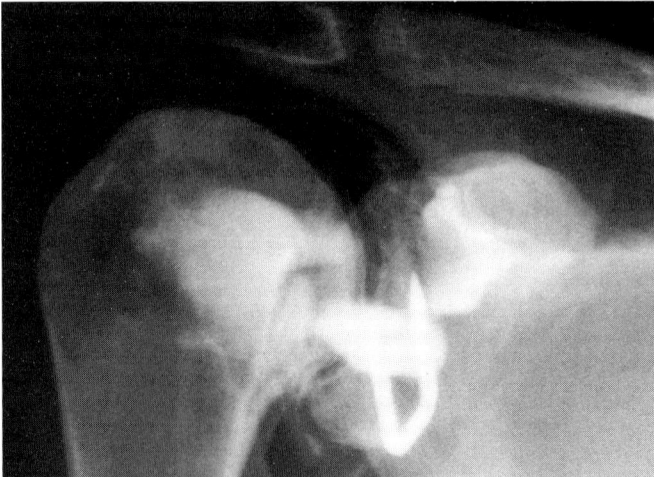

FIGURE 82
Patient with multidirectional instability and persistent inferior instability following a capsulorrhaphy and subscapularis transfer (Magnuson-Stack). **Left,** The patient still has a persistent sulcus sign from a previous surgery. **Right,** An arthrogram showing a persistent inferior pouch despite an anterior repair involving a staple capsulorrhaphy as well as transfer of the subscapularis muscle.

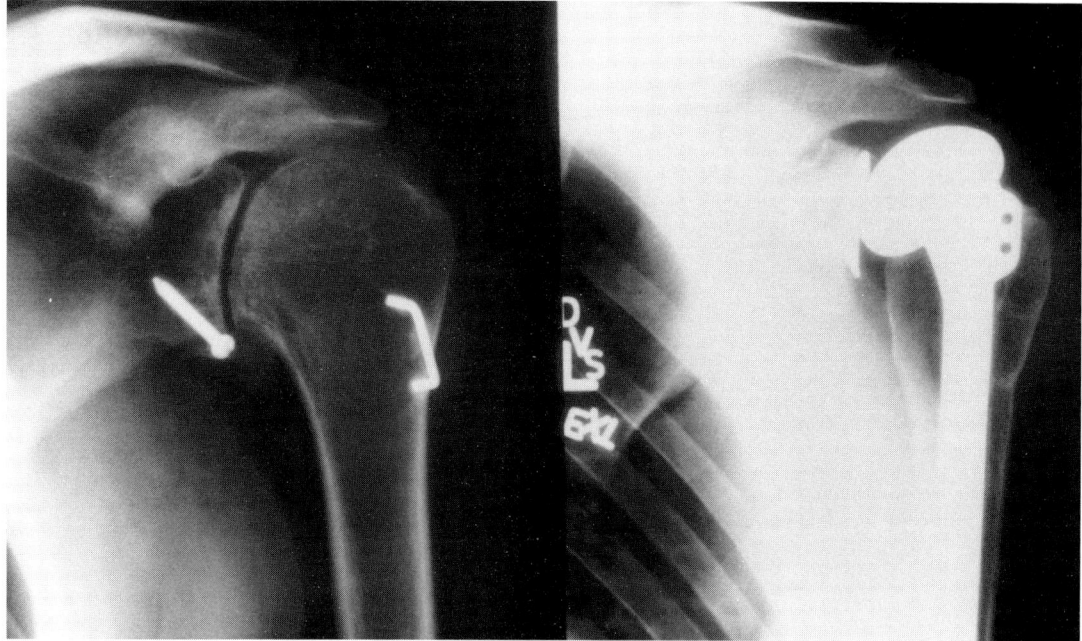

FIGURE 83
Preoperative **(left)** and postoperative **(right)** radiographs of a 58-year-old patient who developed degenerative arthritis following multiple surgeries to the shoulder. The patient required a total shoulder replacement to restore congruity to the joint and relieve pain with improved function.

of the joint. If the rotator interval is closed too tight, the head can be pushed inferiorly (Fig. 82).

If an anterior repair was made too tight, the contractures should be released to equalize the tension across the humeral joints. MacDonald and associates[8] reported on 10 shoulders having internal rotation contractures following anterior repair treated by release of the subscapularis. In addition, six shoulders had radiographic changes of osteoarthritis. After release, all patients had less pain and an average increase of 27° of external rotation. Lusardi and associates[10] reported improvement in pain and range of motion in 20 patients having anterior soft-tissue contractures. Sixteen of these patients had arthritis, with nine requiring prosthetic replacement.

Bigliani and associates[7] reported on 17 patients who had anterior soft-tissue release and prosthetic replacement (12 with total replacement, five with humeral head replacement) with 13 patients (77%) having satisfactory results (Fig. 83). However, 16 patients (94%) achieved adequate pain relief. Excessive soft-tissue scarring and muscle damage

were factors leading to weakness and stiffness in the unsatisfactory results.

Loose or malpositioned hardware should be removed as part of the reconstructive procedure. Young and Rockwood[5] has reported that Bristow procedures are especially difficult to reconstruct; only 50% of the patients in their series had satisfactory results following a revision of a failed Bristow procedure. In this situation there is usually excessive scarring with deformity of the soft tissues secondary to the transfer of the coracoid and conjoined tendons through the subscapularis. This is predominantly an extra-articular repair and there may be residual capsular laxity or a Bankart lesion that has not been repaired.

In conclusion, patients who have failed instability repairs are a complex clinical problem to evaluate. There are often multiple factors present that contribute to the failure of their instability repair. A thorough evaluation is essential with a complete history, physical examination, and radiographic evaluation. The primary goal of surgical repair is to identify and correct the pathology found so that normal anatomy may be restored. However, the results of surgical repair are not as good as primary instability repairs. There should be a high suspicion for the possibility of a voluntary component to the instability. In patients with severe degenerative change in the glenohumeral joint, a prosthesis may be an option to relieve pain and restore function.

REFERENCES

1. Hawkins RH, Hawkins RJ: Failed anterior reconstruction for shoulder instability. *J Bone Joint Surg* 1985;67B:709-714.

2. Hawkins RJ, Angelo RL: Glenohumeral osteoarthrosis: A late complication of the Putti-Platt repair. *J Bone Joint Surg* 1990;72A: 1193-1197.

3. Norris TR, Bigliani LU: Analysis of failed repair for shoulder instability: A preliminary report, in Bateman JE, Welsh RP (eds): *Surgery of the Shoulder*. Philadelphia, PA, BC Decker, 1984, pp 111-116.

4. Rowe CR, Zarins B, Ciullo JV: Recurrent anterior dislocation of the shoulder after surgical repair: Apparent causes of failure and treatment. *J Bone Joint Surg* 1984;66A:159-168.

5. Young DC, Rockwood CA Jr: Complications of a failed Bristow procedure and their management: Apparent causes of failure and treatment. *J Bone Joint Surg* 1991;73A:969-981.

6. Zuckerman JD, Matsen FA III: Complications about the glenohumeral joint related to the use of screws and staples. *J Bone Joint Surg* 1984;66A:175-180.

7. Bigliani LU, Weinstein DM, Glasgow M, et al: Glenohumeral arthroplasty for arthritis after instability surgery. *J Shoulder Elbow Surg* 1995;4:87-94.

8. MacDonald PB, Hawkins RJ, Fowler PJ, et al: Release of the subscapularis for internal rotation contracture and pain after anterior repair for recurrent anterior dislocation of the shoulder. *J Bone Joint Surg* 1992;74A:734-737.

9. O'Driscoll SW, Evans DC: Long-term results of staple capsulorrhaphy for anterior instability of the shoulder. *J Bone Joint Surg* 1993;75A: 249-258.

10. Lusardi DA, Wirth MA, Wurtz D, et al: Loss of external rotation following anterior capsulorrhaphy of the shoulder. *J Bone Joint Surg* 1993;75A:1185-1192.

11. Hovelius L, Akermark C, Albrektsson B, et al: Bristow-Latarjet procedure for recurrent anterior dislocation of the shoulder: A 2-5 year follow-up study on the results of 112 cases. *Acta Orthop Scand* 1983;54:284-290.

12. Flatow EL, Bigliani LU, April EW: An anatomic study of the musculocutaneous nerve and its relationship to the coracoid process. *Clin Orthop* 1989;244:166-171.

13. Richards RR, Hudson AR, Bertoia JT, et al: Injury to the brachial plexus during Putti-Platt and Bristow procedures: A report of eight cases. *Am J Sports Med* 1987;15:374-380.

14. Norris TR: Analysis of instability in 60 shoulders: Diagnostic methods and operative treatment with a capsular shift approach. *Orthop Trans* 1984;8:405.

POSTOPERATIVE REHABILITATION

JAMES E. TIBONE, MD

Rehabilitation after instability surgery is as important as the surgery itself. Without a proper postoperative shoulder rehabilitation program, a well-performed surgery may have a poor outcome. The rehabilitation program must be individualized, although certain guidelines can be followed.

The surgeon and therapist must know which capsular structures and ligaments are stressed with the shoulder in different positions and which muscles are challenged with certain exercises. Exercises performed in the coronal plane of the body will have a different effect on structures than exercises done in the scapular plane of the body. The type of surgical repair, the quality of the repair, and the tightness of the repair all affect the postoperative rehabilitation prescription. Only the surgeon knows these parameters, and he or she must determine them exactly at the time of surgery. For example, in performing an anterior capsular repair of the shoulder, the surgeon should determine at the conclusion of the repair what degree of external rotation stresses the repair by putting a finger on the joint while externally rotating the shoulder to feel the tension on the repair. This test should be done with the patient's arm at the side and also at the 90° elevated position. The results can help determine what amount of external rotation is within the safe zone. If tension develops in the anterior capsule with 30° of external rotation while the arm is at the side, the therapist must be informed that only exercises up to this amount of external rotation should be allowed in the initial phase of therapy. The surgeon must communicate with the therapist so that early stretching or disruption of the repair does not occur because of an aggressive physical therapy program.

Postoperative rehabilitation starts with obtaining range of motion with a proper scapuloglenoid rhythm. Rehabilitation then proceeds to a strengthening program of the rotator cuff, deltoid, and scapular rotator muscles, followed by a program for the power muscles about the shoulders,

the pectoralis major and latissimus dorsi. Finally, a functional program is developed to re-establish proprioception and muscular coordination.

Four major surgical patient groups require different postoperative rehabilitation programs. Group 1 includes the overhead athlete with an anterior capsular repair, such as an anterior capsulolabral reconstruction. Group 2 includes individuals who have undergone an anterior repair for traumatic anterior instability. Group 3 includes individuals who have undergone a posterior capsular repair for posterior instability. Group 4 includes those individuals who have undergone an anterior inferior capsular shift for multidirectional instability.

THE OVERHEAD ATHLETE

The following protocol is based on the work of Brewster and associates.[1]

The initial phase following surgery focuses on decreasing postoperative pain and swelling and achieving full ROM. ROM exercises are started on the first day following surgery. Initially, the patient is immobilized for 1 to 2 weeks in an abduction pillow or brace, with the glenohumeral joint positioned in the plane of the scapula with 90° elevation and 45° external rotation. The orthosis is removed to perform the exercises. A sling with the arm comfortably positioned at the side also may be used. The amount of external rotation allowed initially is determined at the time of surgery. Gentle range of motion is performed twice daily, including internal and external rotation, abduction and adduction, and shoulder flexion. External rotation, internal rotation, and elevation are conducted in the scapular plane. Extension of the shoulder is avoided to protect the capsular repair. ROM should be gentle and should not cause significant pain. Hand and elbow exercises using a soft sponge or ball are started.

Isometric strengthening exercises can also be initiated within the first week following surgery. They are performed in all planes of motion and at multiple angles as tolerated by the athlete.

At 2 weeks following surgery, active/assistive exercises are continued, to increase ROM. Gentle resistive rotation exercises at the side are performed with light theraband or surgical tubing and resistance is gradually increased over a 2- to 3-week period. A towel or the opposite extremity can be placed between the body and the arm to move the shoulder into slight forward flexion, which decreases the stress on the shoulder. At 4 weeks, active elevation in the sagittal plane is added to begin strengthening of the anterior deltoid; resistance is gradually increased over a 2-week period. A goal in an athletic population is to obtain full range of motion by 6 to 8 weeks postoperatively, except for the terminal few degrees of external rotation in the throwing position.

At 4 weeks following surgery, external rotation in a side-lying position is started with light weights (1 to 3 lb). These exercises are done with the arm in the full internal rotation position with external rotation to the neutral position. The patient is started on the upper extremity bicycle to increase strength and endurance.

Glenohumeral motion and scapulothoracic rhythm must be established. The tightness of the scapular muscles will affect ROM and shoulder kinematics. The medial scapular muscles can become tight after shoulder surgery. These must be stretched for proper rotation of the scapula. Rhomboid stretches should be instituted if any tightness is noticed. The rhomboids can be stretched by grabbing onto a door handle with the shoulders forward flexed and leaning back so that the arms are supporting the weight of the body (Fig. 84).

By 2 months following surgery, when full ROM has been obtained, emphasis is placed on strengthening the rotator cuff muscles. Also, increasing stress is applied to the deltoid by allowing shoulder flexion and abduction exercises to 180° rather than 90°.

At 3 months following surgery, isokinetic conditioning can begin. This is done with rotation exercises at the side at fast speeds greater than 200° per second. Slower speeds should not be used as they put too much stress on the shoulder and can lead to an increase in shoulder pain.

Six months postoperatively, isokinetic testing

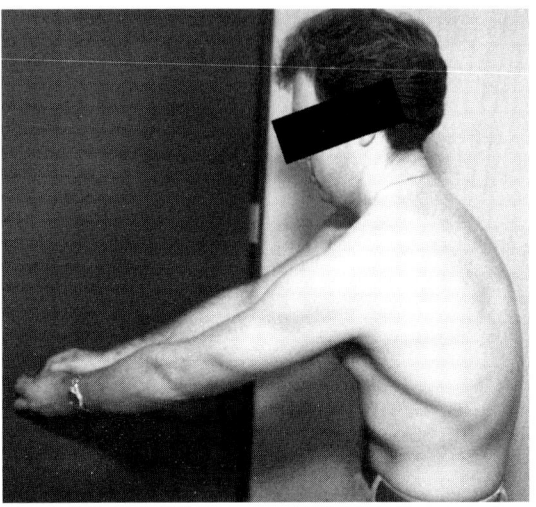

FIGURE 84
Rhomboid stretch.

should reveal 90% of strength on the operated extremity compared to the contralateral side. When this occurs, a throwing program can begin and be performed every other day. If there is any increase in pain or swelling, the throwing program is delayed further. Throwing is begun at half speed and is not progressed to three-quarter speed until 7 to 8 months postoperatively. At 12 months, throwing is allowed at full speed.

Sometimes it may be difficult to make the transition from muscle strengthening exercises to the overhead throwing motion. Overhead medicine ball exercises may provide a useful bridge between strengthening exercises and the dynamic overhead throwing motion. The operated shoulder stimulates the throwing motion but is protected because the contralateral arm is also used. Recent EMG studies of the two-handed overhead medicine ball have revealed similar muscle activity to the throwing motion. Therefore, muscle strength and functional coordination can be developed in a dynamic but relatively safe environment.

It is essential that an athlete obtain full external rotation before returning to competitive overhead sport. This can be accomplished by a surgery that does not overly tighten the capsule, by beginning early ROM, and by establishing strength and flexibility of the rotator cuff and scapular rotator muscles and tendons.

REHABILITATION FOLLOWING ANTERIOR REPAIR FOR TRAUMATIC INSTABILITY

Patients who have anterior repair for traumatic instability can be prone to postoperative stiffness.[1-3] Immobilization in the past was prescribed in this group of patients for 3 to 6 weeks. This is no longer necessary or indicated. Following surgery, the arm is placed in a sling for 2 to 3 weeks for comfort only. The patient is encouraged to remove the sling to perform hand and elbow exercises and to start shoulder motion. The shoulder is elevated in forward flexion and in the scapular plane using pulleys and wands. The therapist performs passive ROM including external rotation in the safe zone, which has been determined by the surgeon at the time of surgical repair and communicated to the physical therapist or trainer. Ice is used to control pain and swelling.

Between 4 and 6 weeks postoperatively, external rotation exercises can be done in the elevated position of 45°, again with the shoulder in the plane of the scapula. Active and active/assistive ROM are used to strengthen the deltoid, rotator cuff, and scapular muscles. The anterior capsule is protected from stretch. Posterior glides, and towel stretches are allowed to stretch out the tight posterior structures. Shoulder shrugs and wall push-ups are performed to strengthen the scapular rotators. Prone rowing and hyperextension exercises are helpful to strengthen the rhomboids and trapezius muscles. The therapist must concentrate on establishing scapulohumeral rhythm, which should return to normal at 12 weeks following surgery.

At 3 months after surgery, full elevation and internal rotation should be achieved, with a loss of 5° to 10° of external rotation compared to the "normal shoulder." At this junction, therapy is used to regain full strength and endurance in the shoulder. Following a traumatic shoulder instability with a subsequent repair, it is not uncommon to lose 10° of external rotation with the arm in the throwing position. Stretching to obtain these last few degrees may be difficult and cause the patient an increase of shoulder pain and therefore should be performed with caution.

Some therapists believe that upper extremity patterns are important in establishing full function in the shoulder. This is called proprioceptive neuromuscular facilitation (PNF).[2] Such patterns can be performed with pulleys or on kinetic machines. This can help in establishing the coordination of the various shoulder movements and muscles.

A continued program is used to maintain strength in the rotator cuff, deltoid, and scapular rotators, as well as the power muscles, the pectoralis major and latissimus dorsi. A core exercise program has been designed to provide an efficient exercise program for the shoulder.[4-6] This includes shoulder flexion for the anterior deltoid (Fig. 85), shoulder elevation in the scapular plane for the supraspinatus (Fig. 86), prone abduction with external rotation for the infraspinatus and teres minor (Fig. 87), a press-up for the pectoralis major and latissimus dorsi (Fig. 88), a push up plus for the serratus anterior (Fig. 89), and horizontal rowing for the trapezius, levator scapulae, and rhomboids (Fig. 90). Elevation in the scapular plane should be done in external rotation. If this exercise is performed in internal rotation as initially recommended, impingement and/or tendinitis may occur.

At 4 months postoperatively, functional exercises can begin, concentrating on sports-specific activity. By 6 months following surgery, a return to sports and full activities is possible.

REHABILITATION FOLLOWING POSTERIOR CAPSULAR REPAIR

The following protocol is based on Tibone and Bradley[7] and Tibone.[8]

Posterior instability is usually secondary to stretching of the posterior capsule and has a higher failure rate of repair than its anterior counterpart.[7,9,10] For this reason, the shoulder is usually immobilized following repair of the posterior capsule. To take the stress off the repair, the shoulder should be kept in extension and slight external rotation. This can be accomplished with an abduction pillow (Fig. 91) or a "gunslinger" orthosis. Immobilization is continued for 4 to 5 weeks with essentially no shoulder exercises. At 4 to 5 weeks after surgery, the upper extremity is removed from the pillow or orthosis and brought down to the side. Full internal rotation should be avoided immediately because this may place too much stress across the repair. External rotation exercises are started at the side. Elevation is begun in the

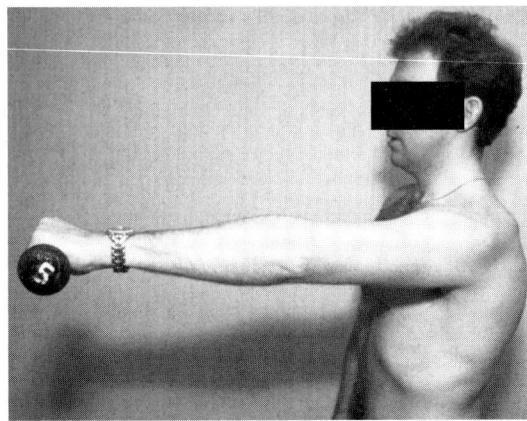

FIGURE 85
Shoulder flexion for deltoid.

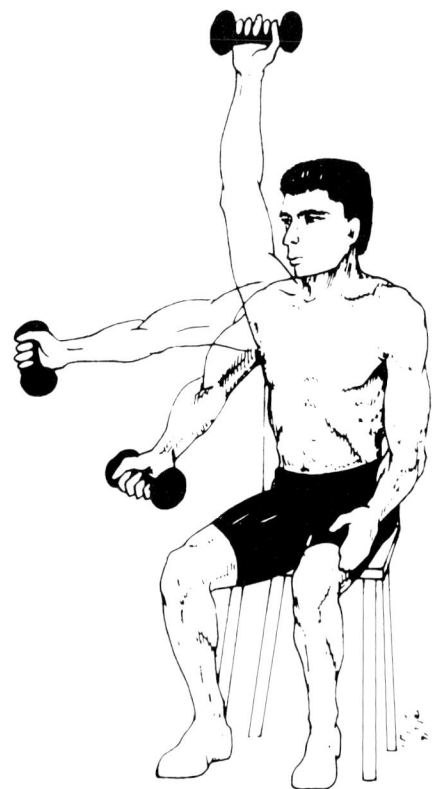

FIGURE 86
Scaption (thumbs up) with external rotation.

scapular plane of the body. No elevation is allowed in the sagittal plane (forward flexion). Forward flexion with internal rotation is not permitted for the first 6 weeks postoperatively. Isometric exercises are begun at 4 weeks in all planes and the internal rotators of the shoulder are slowly stretched. Active and active/assistive external rotation is also important at this stage.

At 6 weeks after surgery, the shoulder can be elevated in the scapular plane in neutral or slight external rotation. ROM exercises at this time are performed without weights. Therabands can be used for resistance exercises to strengthen the rotator cuff and deltoid muscles. Only at 12 weeks after surgery are light weights begun in the rehabilitation program. The emphasis at this time is on the external rotators, the infraspinatus and teres minor. The posterior deltoid is also rehabilitated by performing shoulder elevation in extension exercises. An important exercise for these posterior shoulder muscles is prone abduction with the shoulder in external rotation (Fig. 88). If there is residual stiffness this exercise may be difficult and prone rowing and hyperextension exercises may be more appropriate.

There is no attempt to establish full range of motion quickly. Rehabilitation must be slower than for anterior instability surgery to avoid overly stretching the posterior capsule repair. There is no attempt to obtain full elevation before 3 months postoperatively and, commonly, full ROM may not be established until 6 months. Following posterior instability surgery and after a proper rehabilitation program it is not uncommon to lose two to four spinal levels of internal rotation. This should not be a concern and is probably necessary to maintain stability after a posterior shoulder repair.

No attempt is made to use heavy weights or equipment for 6 months following surgery. Bench presses and push-ups are to be avoided. A full return to sports is delayed for 9 months. A throwing athlete can usually start to throw at 9 months, but competitive throwing takes a minimum of 1 year. Some posterior instability patients also have abnormal shoulder kinematics. The scapula may have some amount of winging during the rehabilitation process. Rehabilitation must concentrate on establishing the proper scapulohumeral rhythm and retraining the serratus anterior and trapezius to function in a normal pattern.

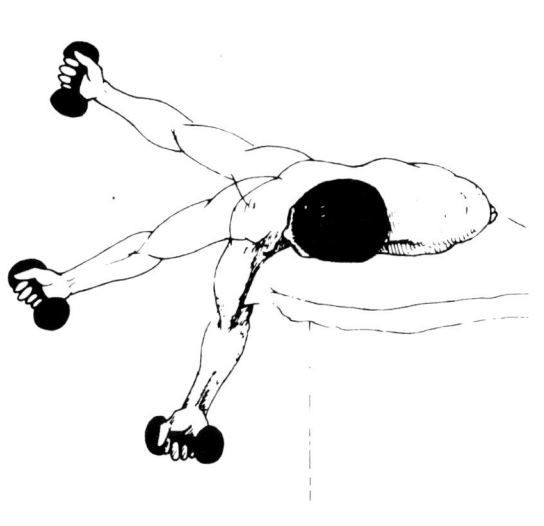

FIGURE 87
Horizontal abduction in external rotation.

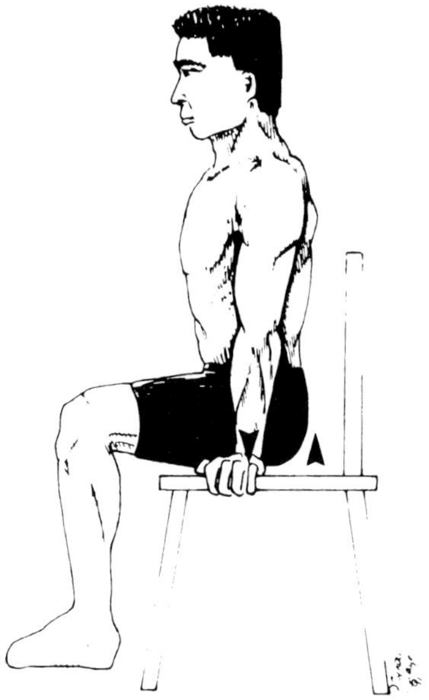

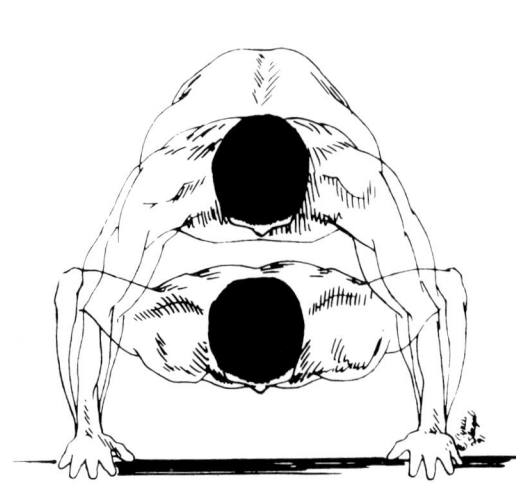

FIGURE 89
Push-up plus.

FIGURE 88
Press-up.

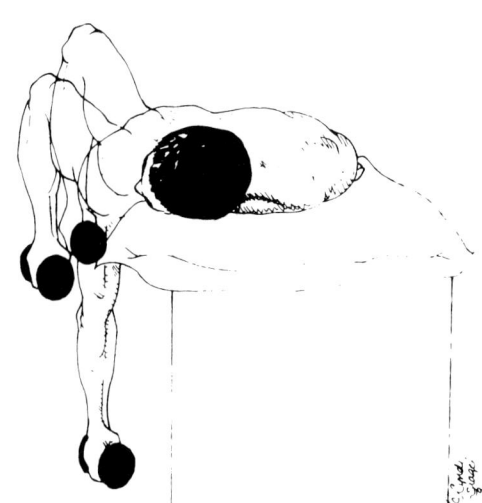

FIGURE 90
Rowing.

REHABILITATION FOLLOWING SURGERY FOR MULTIDIRECTIONAL INSTABILITY

The following protocol is based on the work of Cordasco and associates.[11]

Patients with true multidirectional instability are a difficult surgical and rehabilitation problem.[12] These loose-jointed individuals should be immobilized for a minimum of 6 weeks with no motion exercises. Immobilization can be accomplished in a sling if the main multidirectional component is anterior and inferior. If there is a significant posterior component to the multidirectional instability, then the patient should be immobilized in an orthosis with the arm at the side held in neutral rotation. The only exercises allowed at this time are for the wrist and hand.

Following 6 weeks of immobilization, exercises are started. With multidirectional instability, no passive exercises are needed. Some limitation of motion at the end of rehabilitation is desirable, and the therapist must be instructed to proceed slowly. These patients have no problem stretching out their capsule and regaining most of their motion. They commonly have poor shoulder musculature and poor control of their shoulder. Passive exercises are started initially and quickly advance to active/assistive and active exercises to develop muscle control. Light theraband is used for resistance and gradually increased.

Light weights are begun at 3 months. These patients commonly can only start with weights between 1 and 3 lb and have difficulty regaining their strength. Emphasis should be placed on increased repetitions rather than on dramatic

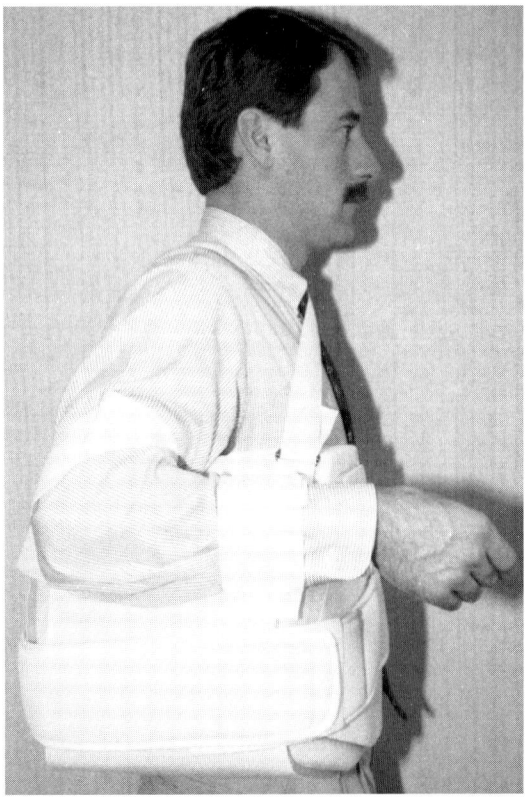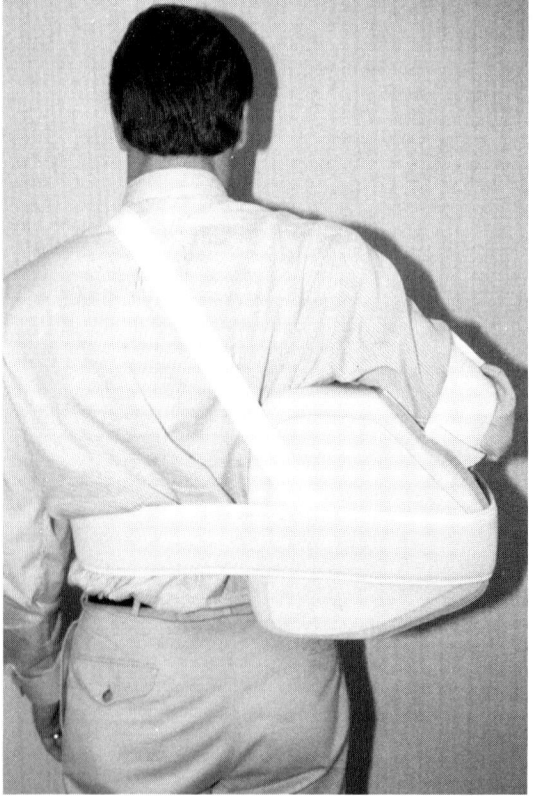

FIGURE 91
The postoperative abduction pillow is shown with the shoulder in slight extension and neutral rotation.

increases in weight. The scapular rotator muscles are commonly weak and need to be retrained. These patients are also prone to "tendinitis" that slows down the rehabilitation progress. They need to be followed very closely and managed with proper anti-inflammatory medications and ice.

Any return to sports is not recommended for 1 year; for the nonathlete, satisfactory function is usually not obtained for 1 year.

CONCLUSION

Rehabilitation following shoulder instability surgery requires that the surgeon document the tightness of the repair in different shoulder positions at the time of surgery. Significant immobilization usually is not needed after anterior surgery in overhead athletes or individuals with traumatic anterior instability. Patients with posterior instability or multidirectional instability usually have significant capsular stretching that will benefit from 3 to 6 weeks of immobilization postoperatively.

When exercises are begun, range of motion is the primary concern, followed by reestablishment of scapulothoracic and glenohumeral rhythm. Strengthening is then started on the rotator cuff and scapular rotator muscles. Rehabilitation of the deltoid muscle is next emphasized, followed by regaining strength of the power muscles (pectoralis major, latissimus dorsi) of the shoulder. Finally, for the athlete, a functional program is started to regain coordination, proprioception, and sports-related activity.

As with any shoulder surgery, without proper rehabilitation, the result will be less than optimal. Awareness of the proper postoperative rehabilitation program is therefore mandatory for orthopaedic surgeons.

REFERENCES

1. Brewster CE, Seto JL, Moynes DR, et al: Capsulolabral reconstruction and rehabilitation, in Andrews JR, Wilk KE (eds): *The Athlete's Shoulder.* New York, NY, Churchill Livingstone, 1994, pp 221-229.

2. Kennedy K: Rehabilitation of the unstable shoulder. *Oper Tech Sports Med* 1993;1:331-324.

3. Wilk KE, Arrigo C: Current concepts in the rehabilitation of the athletic shoulder. *J Orthop Sports Phys Ther* 1993;18:365-378.

4. Townsend H, Jobe FW, Pink M, et al: Electromyographic analysis of the glenohumeral muscles during a baseball rehabilitation program. *Am J Sports Med* 1991;19:264-272.

5. Moseley JB Jr, Jobe FW, Pink M, et al: EMG analysis of the scapular muscles during a shoulder rehabilitation program. *Am J Sports Med* 1992;20:128-134.

6. Bradley JP, Tibone JE: Electromyographic analysis of muscle action about the shoulder. *Clin Sports Med* 1991;10:789-805.

7. Tibone JE, Bradley JP: The treatment of posterior subluxation in athletes. *Clin Orthop* 1993;291:124-137.

8. Tibone JE: Posterior capsulorrhaphy for posterior shoulder subluxation, in Paulos LE, Tibone JE (eds): *Operative Techniques in Shoulder Surgery.* Gaithersburg, MD, Aspen Publishers, 1991, pp 143-147.

9. Hawkins RJ, Koppert G, Johnston G: Recurrent posterior instability (subluxation) of the shoulder. *J Bone Joint Surg* 1984;66A:169-174.

10. Tibone J, Ting A: Capsulorrhaphy with a staple for recurrent posterior subluxation of the shoulder. *J Bone Joint Surg* 1990;72A:999-1002.

11. Cordasco FA, Pollock RG, Flatow EL, et al: Management of multidirectional instability. *Op Tech in Sports Med* 1993;1:293-300.

12. Neer CS II, Foster CR: Inferior capsular shift for involuntary inferior and multidirectional instability of the shoulder: A preliminary report. *J Bone Joint Surg* 1980;62A:897-908.

INDEX